AIDS in Jewish Thought and Law

Edited and with an introduction by

Gad Freudenthal

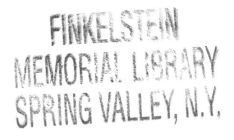
KTAV Publishing House, Inc.

1998

Library of Congress Cataloging-in-Publication Data

Freudenthal, Gad.
    AIDS in Jewish Thought and Law / edited and with an introduction by
Gad Freudenthal.
        p.   cm.
    Includes bibliographical references and index.
    ISBN 0-88125-610-2 (hc)
    1. AIDS (Disease)—Religious aspects—Judaism.   2. Medicine—Religious
aspects—Judaism.   3. Medical laws and legislation (Jewish law)   4. Ethics, Jewish.
5. Medical ethics.   I. Freudenthal, Gad.
BM538.H43J49   1998
296.3'8—dc21   96-36232
                                                                                                    CIP

Manufactured in the United States of America
KTAV Publishing House, Inc.
900 Jefferson St.
Hoboken, NJ 07030

Contents

Preface

Like any novel societal phenomenon, the Acquired Immunodeficiency Syndrome (AIDS) pandemic, which gradually entered public consciousness in the early 1980s, forced Jewish thinkers—rabbis, physicians, philosophers, and others—to consider whether this scourge raises new issues or problems for Judaism. The present volume is intended to provide a fairly full picture of the Jewish responses to AIDS, notably in the United States of America, the United Kingdom, Israel, and France. The volume consists of my own Introduction, followed by practically all the major texts of which I am aware bearing on the subject of AIDS and Judaism;[1] also included are all the published responsa on issues related to AIDS (as it happens, they are all Reform responsa). To avoid misunderstandings, let me emphasize that my interest is not in how various Jewish communities have confronted AIDS on the practical level of social action, but in theological and halakhic reflections on issues related to AIDS. Nonetheless, to make this volume as informative and useful as possible, some official statements on AIDS by various Jewish bodies are also included.

All the texts are reproduced with only minor stylistic systematization (done by the publisher), as well as occasional corrections of typographical errors and some systematization of Hebrew transliterations, etc. (The only exception is Rav

Deichowsky's article, whose English translation has been thoroughly revised by the editor.)* Information on initial publication of the texts, and related matters, will be found in the Acknowledgments section. The bibliographic references in the notes have been systematized to some extent, but authors' deliberate preferences (e.g., between "God" and "G-d," "divine" and "Divine") have been scrupulously respected.

A note on my own stance in compiling the volume, and specifically in writing the Introduction, is in order. The writers represented or discussed in this volume typically examine this or that question in an effort to determine what is right and what is wrong from the viewpoint of Judaism: theirs is a *normative* stance. Not being a rabbi or an expert on Halakhah, my own position is different, and the Introduction, too, belongs to a different literary genre: my stance is deliberately *descriptive*—it is that of the scholar, the historian of ideas or of religion, whose raw material consists of the normative pronouncements on AIDS and Judaism made by others. The reprinting of the articles and the Introduction thus follow the goal of providing an accurate and full picture of the views and opinions on issues related to AIDS that have been expressed within Judaism since 1986, when the first statements on AIDS were made by Jewish authors. The Introduction, specifically, does not enunciate any normative positions; I simply discuss the opinions of various authors and juxtapose them, here and there pausing to interject a comment, to draw the reader's attention to some underlying premises of the argument, or to compare the arguments adduced on a given issue by different authors.

It is truly a pleasure for me to acknowledge with gratitude the debts I have incurred while preparing this book. First and foremost, I am very much indebted to all the authors who kindly agreed to the inclusion of their writings in this volume. I am also grateful to the institutions that gave permission for the reprinting of materials for which they hold the copyright. My friends and colleagues Roseline Kalifa (Paris), Menachem Kellner (Haifa

---

• For technical reasons, no diacritical marks could be used in the transliteration of Hebrew words. Thus *h* stands for both *he* and *het*, *z* for both *zadi* and *zayin*, etc. We trust that the reader knowledgeable of Hebrew will supply the missing information him or herself, while for other readers the distinction is anyway meaningless.

University), Josef Stern (University of Chicago), and Hava Tirosh-Samuelson (University of Indiana) were very helpful and supportive both intellectually and practically. Many individuals responded patiently and in detail to my queries concerning their, or their movements', views on AIDS. May they all find here the expression of my hearty thanks.

In France, my tenure at the Centre National de la Recherche Scientifique (CNRS) allowed me to initiate myself into a subject of which at the outset I knew next to nothing. The government-sponsored Agence Nationale de Recherches sur le Sida (ANRS) created adequate conditions for my research by supporting it with a generous grant during the years 1994–1995. I am sincerely grateful to both institutions.

I dedicate this volume to the dear memory of my mother, Renate Freudenthal née Engel (Berlin, 27 July 1910–Jerusalem, 28 October 1997), תנצב"ה.

G.F.

Paris
July 1996

Notes

1. The only notable (and very regrettable) exception is J. David Bleich, "AIDS: A Jewish Perspective," *Tradition* 26, no. 3 (1992): 49–80, which unfortunately we were not authorized to reprint.

ABBREVIATIONS

AIDS	Acquired Immunodeficiency Syndrome
HIV	Human Immunodeficiency Virus
PWA	Person with AIDS
PWHIV	Person with HIV Infection

Introduction

ℵ

Gad Freudenthal

The AIDS pandemic confronted Judaism with a number of novel problems and issues. There were, first and foremost, the practical problems of how to assist AIDS sufferers and people who have contracted HIV.[1] With these, however, we will not be concerned here.[2] The sudden appearance of the pandemic also raised a number of intellectual issues: some were purely theoretical, in fact theological, and related to possible spiritual interpretations AIDS can receive within Judaism; others were matters of Halakhah, bearing on practical matters of conduct. It is these two clusters of problems that will be at the core of our attention in what follows.

One may well begin by wondering why AIDS became the subject of such detailed and specific attention: is it not a malady like any other, even if it qualifies as an epidemic? What is singular about AIDS that allows one to speak of a "Jewish response" to AIDS, whereas no one would think of seeking a Jewish response to cancer or to cardiovascular diseases? The answer obviously lies in the perceived link between AIDS and homosexuality and drug abuse, as well as in the concrete historical setting within which AIDS appeared and which shaped the responses to the pandemy in society at large.

From the outset, AIDS and homosexuality were very closely associated in the public perception. When AIDS appeared in the early 1980s, at first spreading mainly among homosexuals and intravenous drug users, it was naturally perceived as the "gay disease." (This fact, incidentally, brought in its sequel a fairly long delay in the reaction of the Reagan administration to the pandemic.)[3] Now, the decade preceding the appearance of AIDS had witnessed a profound change in the societal standing of homosexuality: in the 1970s, homosexuals increasingly "came out of the closet" and, moreover, demanded that society recognize them as a *community* having its own particular "way of life." In the United States especially, where other "minorities" too had seen their specific demands increasingly granted, the late 1970s witnessed the constitution of "gays" as a distinct community which insisted on its being viewed as a social group with its own lifestyle.

This development was vehemently opposed within Judaism, mainly by its Orthodox and Conservative branches. In fact, from the Jewish perspective, the gays' demand that their sexual preferences be recognized as an alternative lifestyle meant that where beforehand there had been individual sinners who could be tolerated as such—just as there are persons not respecting Shabbat or *kashrut*—there was now a self-conscious *group* defining itself essentially by reference to a practice that had been considered to be an abomination. Moreover, as has been pointed out by Rabbi Alan Unterman, whereas sins usually are incidental to the sinner's identity, gays *define* themselves specifically with reference to their sin, their sexual identity being "constitutive of their very identity."[4] This gay attitude, let us note, is clearly an aspect of modernity, inasmuch as it is an integral part of the conception that the autonomy of the individual includes his or her right to sexual self-fulfillment. The confrontation between the gays' demands and the positions of traditional Judaism should therefore be viewed as an aspect of the confrontation between the traditional values of Judaism and modernity.

Christian denominations too, as a rule, strongly resented the social legitimation of homosexuality in the United States.[5] When AIDS appeared in the early 1980s, some conservative religious thinkers, mainly Christian fundamentalist preachers, felt it was a divine response to the homosexuals' effrontery in the preceding decade. *Qua* a disease hitting mainly a group of people whose own self-definition was based on the transgression of a divine commandment, AIDS from the outset appeared to have a singular religious status; by virtue of its connection with homosexuality, AIDS seemed *ipso facto* to acquire a theological dimension.

Now questions concerning divine retribution through illnesses are a *topos* that is not new to Judaism, and it is therefore little wonder that several authors have addressed the question whether AIDS should be construed as a divine punishment of homosexuality. These discussions are studied in the first part of the Introduction.

In addition to the theological problem, AIDS raises some specific halakhic problems, which are the subject of the second part of the Introduction. Some of these problems are again related to the pandemic's association with homosexuality and drug abuse. Thus, the question has come up whether, according to Halakhah, persons with HIV and persons with AIDS (in what follows: PWHIVs and PWAs, respectively)[6] should be provided with medical care. As is well known, Judaism accords great importance to the precept of visiting and assisting the sick, and it is thus surprising to find that the issue is even a subject for discussion. The reason for this is simply that from the Jewish perspective (just as from the Christian or the Moslem one), most AIDS sufferers are simultaneously sick and sinners,[7] and the question can be raised whether the precept of caring for the sick applies to someone who contracted an illness as a result of a behavior that constitutes a transgression of a divine commandment. Another question on which Halakhah has had to determine its position is that of prevention: state authorities in various countries have launched prevention campaigns promoting "safer sex" and advocating the supply of clean needles to intravenous drug users, and Jewish authors had to evaluate these measures from the vantage point of Halakhah. Lastly, Jewish authors also had to take a stand on issues much debated by secular thinkers and related to the balance which policy makers must strike between the restrictive and coercive measures called for by public health policy and the criteria of individual human rights, which usually are incompatible with any coercive measures. Thus, Jewish authors had to consider the position of Halakhah on such issues as mandatory screening for AIDS and confidentiality regarding information on one's serological status.

The Theological Problematic: AIDS a Divine Retribution?

We neither can nor need go here into a review of the attitudes toward homosexuality expressed within Judaism. Suffice it to say that with the rise of the gay movement, a number of Jewish authors have subjected the traditionally hostile attitude of Judaism toward homosexuality to new scrutiny. It is in this context, it seems, that Rabbi Norman Lamm put forward the innovative suggestion to view at least some homosexuals as suffering from a malady and therefore as acting under compulsion (*ones*), with the consequence that whereas the act itself remains a transgression, "the person who transgresses is considered innocent on grounds of *ones*."[8] However, this option has not been accepted, nor even seriously considered, by the halakhic writers[9] who have written on AIDS and whom we will consider here.[10] These writers are unanimous in viewing homosexual acts as an abomination explicitly forbidden by the Bible.[11] The use of drugs too—even of marijuana and *a fortiori* of hard drugs injected intravenously—is forbidden, mainly on the grounds that it endangers the user.[12] The appreciation of homosexual behavior and of drug abuse is thus not under dispute among the authors under consideration here; the question is how they construe the *relationship* between those transgressions and AIDS. To this we now turn.

Contrary to what might perhaps have been expected, not only within halakhic Judaism but even within Orthodox Judaism, the question concerning the possible theological significance of AIDS received quite different, indeed opposite, answers. The two possible extremes were formulated almost simultaneously at the end of 1986 by Rabbi Barry Freundel in the United States and by Rabbi Immanuel Jakobovits in Great Britain. Whereas the former strongly leans toward the view that AIDS is a divine retribution, the latter from the outset forbids himself to engage in any speculation on the issue.

Rabbi Freundel begins his examination of the question with a sort of epistemological disclaimer: "To the question of AIDS as divine retribution no final answer can be given. We lack a prophet, *Urim we-Tumin,* or *Ruah Ha-Qodesh* to ask the One who knows";[13] indeed, "God's understanding of things is not the same as ours, and, therefore, we can ascribe causality in the divine realm only with great temerity, if at all."[14] Thus, on the epistemological level, Rabbi Freundel's position is, as he puts it, *agnostic.*[15] Freundel also unambiguously states that the issue is of no practical importance: he argues, first, that the theological question of AIDS as a divine retribution came to the fore only because such a claim was made by Christian fundamentalists,[16] and, second, that in any event the stance one takes on this issue must not affect one's practical behavior toward AIDS patients.[17] Yet, notwithstanding his declared epistemological agnosticism and the practical irrelevance of the issue, Freundel scrutinizes in detail the pros and cons of the thesis that AIDS is a divine retribution, and clearly falls in with the pros.

In Freundel's view, "By far, the greater evidence indicates that God's retribution plays a role in epidemics such as AIDS." His argument is this: since several passages in the Bible predict "the land's physical rejection of those guilty of immorality in general, and homosexuality specifically, it does not take a great leap of faith to see the hand of God in the AIDS epidemic."[18] Rabbinic statements like the one affirming that the Flood was brought upon the world because of the sexual immorality of the generation appear to Freundel as "a frightening foreshadowing of the AIDS phenomenon."[19] Such a stance obviously presupposes a view of God as constantly exerting His judgment over each and every detail of every person's moral behavior. This is a view of providence according to which, as Rabbi Freundel formulates it, divine retribution is an "active principle in the universe";[20] Freundel maintains that Rabbinic sources speak of "God arranging events . . . so that those guilty of capital crimes [such as homosexuality, which is a capital crime for Jews and gentiles alike] . . .

will receive the appropriate punishment" even in the absence of a suitable court to sentence them.[21] Freundel discerns in the Bible and the Talmud an "unequivocal belief in the power and contemporary reality of divine retribution," allowing one to conclude that "the vast majority of traditional statements . . . tend to support the 'AIDS as Divine Retribution' theory."[22]

Freundel concedes, however, that the opposite opinion can also claim the support of some textual proofs. The Talmudic statement that "All is in the hands of Heaven, except heat, cold" may be interpreted as bearing on the illnesses that climatic changes may entail.[23] It is therefore arguable that this reasoning can be applied to the case of AIDS, although in Freundel's view this requires "a bit of a stretch."[24] A second consideration pointing in the same direction proceeds on the view of Hazon Ish (Rabbi Avraham Karelitz, 1878–1953) that "divine reward and punishment are not as universally visible today as they once were," so that perhaps after all "God is not merely using AIDS to punish sinners."[25]

Rabbi Freundel's position, let me note in passing, is quite exceptional in the landscape of contemporary Jewish philosophical thought. Throughout its existence, Judaism has witnessed a multitude of views on divine providence: whereas the Bible and many parts of the Talmuds indeed express a generally firm belief in personal providence, this has increasingly been eroded since the time Jewish thought entered into contact with Greek philosophy in the medieval period.[26] (It is therefore significant, and not a mere hazard, that Freundel grounds his position essentially in texts from the earlier periods.) Rabbi Freundel's strong adherence to the belief in personal divine providence is definitely out of step with the views about this issue prevailing among most modern Jewish thinkers (especially after the Holocaust).[27]

Although Rabbi Freundel believes, then, that the question whether AIDS is a divine retribution cannot be settled with certainty, his considered opinion is that "the singling out of the homosexual and drug-user populations as victims of the disease does seem to point to, at the very least, a divine 'cease and desist' order. . . . All involved should examine their deeds and repent for their sins."[28]

A comparable view was expressed by Professor David Novak in 1992. Novak affirms that "AIDS seems to raise what was thought by most moderns to be an ancient superstition long behind us, namely, the whole issue of God's punishment of sin through physical maladies."[29] Novak does not express his own view in unambiguous terms. On the one hand, he seems to distance himself from the "ancient superstition" by situating the connection between sin and AIDS on the level of the *subjective consciousness* of the afflicted persons; he proceeds on the premise that "most of the people in our culture . . . still regard homosexual acts and the use of narcotic drugs to be not only immoral but sinful,"[30] and goes on to affirm that when people learn they are seropositive or have AIDS, it is *they* who, faced with their predicament, perceive a causal connection between their illness and their fault. Novak thus cautiously formulates: "the cultural message about AIDS seems to be that it is caused not only by one's own acts, but by one's immoral or sinful acts";[31] it is not Novak, but rather the afflicted persons themselves, who perceive a causal connection between sin and predicament. On the other hand, however, Novak also uses objectivistic formulations, suggesting that he himself, too, considers AIDS a divine retribution. Thus, children who are born with AIDS appear to him as subsumable under the Biblical principle that children are punished for the sins of their parents and, more generally, under the doctrine of "original sin," which, according to him, Judaism "affirms": "we suffer not only for our own sins but for the sins of others before us."[32] In sum, therefore, "the majority of AIDS sufferers are considered to be in the category of sinners,"[33] and Novak, who wants neither to endorse explicitly the "ancient superstition" nor to reject it, leaves the reader to infer that this is not a mere coincidence. Only in a footnote does he explicitly affirm his belief (strictly identical to Freundel's) that "traditional Jewish theology [emphasizes] that everything other than our own free response to God is indeed 'in the hands of God.'"[34]

As against this intellectual and moral uncertainty (which may be deliberate), the position expressed by Lord Immanuel Jakobovits, then Chief Rabbi of the British Commonwealth, is striking for its moral rectitude and theological soundness; it is indeed without the slightest shadow of ambiguity and is worth being quoted at some length:

> . . . under no circumstances would we be justified in brand-
> ing the incidence of the disease, individually or collectively,
> as punishment that singles out individuals or groups for
> wrongdoing and lets them suffer as a consequence. We are
> not inspired enough, prophetic enough, we have not the
> vision, that would enable us to link, as an assertion of cer-
> tainty, any form of human travail, grief and bereavement or
> suffering in general with shortcomings of a moral nature—
> especially our generation, living as we still do, in the imme-
> diate aftermath of the Holocaust, where millions of Jews
> were done to death with the most unspeakable brutality. We
> certainly should beware of ever identifying specific forms of
> grief, suffering, or anxiety with specific moral or any other
> shortcomings. It is not part of the Jewish doctrine of reward
> and punishment to so identify individual cases with indi-
> vidual experiences of great anguish. I therefore do not go
> along with, but on the contrary, strongly reject and oppose
> those preachers, or would-be preachers, who declare that it
> is Divine vengeance, that the wrath of God is being visited
> on those who deserve it because they live in the cesspools of
> evil.[35]

Rabbi Jakobovits thus follows the principled position of the Hazon Ish and holds that certain ancient authoritative texts, including precisely those adduced by Freundel, can no longer be applied directly and with no interpretive mediation to contemporary situations: the millenary-old events they describe cannot be viewed as unproblematical pertinent precedents. Indeed, he observes that it is inconsistent to subject some scourges (such as AIDS) to moral analysis, but exempt others (earthquakes, floods, or droughts): "There is no such simplistic relationship between evil and misfortune."[36] Rabbi Jakobovits does not dwell at any length on the theological and hermeneutical premises underlying his views, but they are clear enough: whether because of the limits of our understanding ("we are not inspired enough") or a change in God's ways, a literal, immediate application of Scriptural narratives to current situations (Freundel's view of the Flood as a "a frightening foreshadowing of the AIDS phenomenon") is improper. This theological-*cum*-hermeneutic position is the precise antipode of fundamentalism and literalism.

Rabbi Jakobovits suggests an alternative way to construe AIDS and its moral dimension, namely, to view AIDS as a *natural* consequence of certain social practices which happen to be a moral depravity. "There is all the difference—even if the distinction is a fine one—between ascribing massive suffering to personal or social depravity as a divine visitation, and warning that such a depravity may *lead* to terrible consequences."[37] A child who ignores the warning not to play with fire and gets burned is hurt, but this is not a punishment for the disobedience, although it certainly is a consequence thereof. "So there is a clear line of demarcation between punishment and consequence to be drawn."[38] AIDS, then, is a natural consequence of certain forms of life, namely, such that are "morally unacceptable, and utterly repugnant to us."[39] For Rabbi Jakobovits, indeed, AIDS is the *natural* outcome, a *causal* effect, of the violation of a law of nature which is simultaneously also a divine moral law: "we should declare in very plain and explicit terms that our society violated some of the norms of the Divine Law, and of the natural law, and that as a consequence we pay a price, and an exceedingly heavy price."[40] More explicitly still: "AIDS is the price we pay for the 'benefits' of the permissive society which . . . has demolished the last defences of sexual restraint and self-discipline, leading to a collapse of nature's self-defence against degeneracy."[41] Indeed, the violation of the imperatives of sexual morality entails the devastation of the family as a stable social unit, a process whose cost in terms of human misery is even greater than that caused by AIDS.[42] Underlying Rabbi Jakobovits's stance is a view on which the cosmos could—and indeed should—be in a state of harmony, following divine natural-*cum*-moral laws, a harmony that has been jeopardized by certain forms of social, notably sexual, conduct; AIDS is the natural, causal, effect of this disruption of the equilibrium of the cosmos, and it will disappear if and only if the unnatural-*cum*-immoral forms of conduct cease and the harmony of the cosmos is established.

The view of AIDS as resulting from a disruption of the harmony of the cosmos is made explicit and endorsed by Rabbi

Isaac Jessurun of Marseilles. He reports Rabbi Jakobovits's ideas with approval and then goes on to suggest that the primeval, pure and balanced state of the universe is symbolized by the Garden of Eden. Rabbi Jessurun further underscores his vision of AIDS as a disruption of the original equilibrium of the universe with the following metaphor:

> the most surprising fact is that AIDS in fact is not an illness at all: it is a deficiency of the immunological system. The infected person is not "ill," but simply has no more defenses. This confirms our view: society has interfered with the immunological system of the universe, thus damaging the deep-seated structures of Creation.[43]

Dr. Abraham Steinberg holds the very same view: AIDS to him is an "epidemiological-medical justification" of the Jewish stance against homosexuality.[44]

A very similar position is expressed independently by Rabbi J. David Bleich. He, too, opines that "no one, other than a prophet, can declare with certainty that there is a direct cause and effect relationship between a specific misdeed and any particular misfortune."[45] Indeed, Judaism distinguishes between sinners and their sins, and seeks the eradication of sin, not of the sinners.[46] Bleich, too, considers AIDS a natural consequence of certain circumstances, but emphasizes that sinful conduct is only one of them: "Exposure to contagion, whether through transfusion of contaminated blood or sexual intercourse with an infected person, is no different from exposure to extreme heat or cold, in a sense that the resultant disease is the product of man's own folly or negligence."[47] Bleich even goes out of his way to state, *contra* Novak, that "there are countless individuals who have contracted AIDS in a manner which leaves them totally and completely blameless."[48] Yet he too, like Jakobovits, holds that although on the level of the individual, AIDS "may be natural rather than providential," still, since "even the laws of nature are of divine authorship," therefore "it is incumbent upon society to examine the present-day AIDS epidemic in order to determine what can be learnt from it." The lesson Bleich draws from AIDS is, to be sure, much the same as Jakobovits's: "Were our societal standards in conformity with divinely mandated norms the opportunity for individual contagion would simply not arise. In the ultimate sense, every phenomenon is a manifestation of providence. There can be no doubt that it is divinely intended that we take stock of our social standards and practices and realign them in a manner consonant with divine teaching."[49]

As could be expected, Reform Judaism, which in June 1990 adopted a resolution allowing for gay and lesbian rabbis,[50] has rejected from the outset any idea of a possible theological meaning to AIDS. In fact, in June 1986, the Central Conference of American Rabbis took a position on the question and adopted the following resolution:

> We wholly reject the suggestion that has been offered by some, that AIDS may be understood as a special punishment visited by God on a particular class of sinners. AIDS is a viral disease, and, as such, follows natural laws. The difficult theological problem of suffering must be solved for all cases, not dealt with in only those areas where prejudice is substituted for reason or love.[51]

It can easily be recognized that, as far as the theory of divine providence is concerned, this position is strictly identical with that of Rabbi Jakobovits; to be sure, however, there is no word in it paralleling Jakobovits's condemnation of homosexuality as an abomination.

Similarly, a semiofficial opinion expressed in 1987 by Rabbi Joel Roth, chairman of the Committee on Jewish Law and Standards of the United Synagogue of Conservative Judaism, states: "From a halakhic perspective, it is not within the scope of any Jew to make judgments regarding the guilt or 'causes' of illness of any patient (AIDS sufferers or others). Judgments of any type remain in the Divine realm. In any case, not all AIDS patients contract the disease due to objectionable lifestyle."[52]

We may thus conclude, with some satisfaction as far as I am personally concerned, that Jewish authors as a rule straightaway reject, or at least do not hammer out, the notion that AIDS is a divine retribution. Even Novak and Freundel, who clearly incline toward this view, shun away from professing it straightforwardly and without reserve, as Christian fundamentalists do,[53] but rather suggest it cautiously. For most halakhic authors, AIDS is a natural consequence of certain forms of life, and therefore a societal problem; this societal problem is simultaneously a moral and religious problem only because of the contingent fact that the forms of life in question are sinful, so that they disrupt the divine cosmic natural-*cum*-moral order.[54]

Let me mention in passing that the range of opinions found among Jewish writers on the issue of whether AIDS is a divine retribution parallels to a certain extent that observable within the Roman Catholic Church, especially in the United States.[55] On the one hand, the pope has intimated that AIDS is related to sin, although he at the same time unambiguously upholds the more of extending love and help to those afflicted. On the other hand, the California bishops call not only for compassion and for an end to discrimination against persons with HIV and AIDS, but also vigorously reject any attempt to view the disease as a divine manifestation, unambiguously stating that "AIDS must never be considered a divine punishment for a person's sexual orientation, life-style or sexual activity."[56] Other (non-fundamentalist) Christian denominations, too, reject the idea of AIDS as a divine retribution in their official statements.[57]

Another comparative observation is the following. It is interesting to notice that in the Christian tradition the rejection of the idea that AIDS is a divine punishment, and the resulting destigmatization of PWA and PWHIV, follows routes of argumentation paralleling only in part those followed within the Jewish tradition. In the Christian discourse, the notion that AIDS is a divine retribution has been countered, first, by "demythologizing" the disease—arguing that it is a natural outcome of certain biological and social conditions. This, as we have seen, is also the path that has been taken by Jewish thinkers. But arguments of other types proceed on distinctly Christian theological notions not shared by Judaism. Thus, some appeal to "a religious tradition which identifies the sufferer with the suffering servant of God, Jesus Christ," thereby providing "a mythology which would make the AIDS victim bear a special link to Christ"[58]; others proceed from a general image of God as compassionate and commiserative, arguing that it is incompatible with God's nature to use AIDS as a punishment.[59]

Halakhic Problems: The Obligation to Help AIDS Sufferers

We now come to consider the question of how halakhic Judaism construes one's obligations toward the seropositive persons and persons with AIDS. At a first glance, it would seem that no problem can possibly arise here: Judaism famously upholds the duty of visiting and assisting the sick (*biqqur holim*);[60] no less forcefully does it uphold the commandment of trying to save or to prolong life that is at risk.[61] Why should AIDS sufferers be a case apart? Is it not plain that the precepts of *biqqur holim* and of saving one's neighbor's life apply to them just as to any other sick person?

And yet it is a fact that the issue whether PWHIVs and PWAs should be cared for has been discussed at length by Jewish authors; obviously there is something about AIDS that induced them to view this case as singular. The reason is indeed not far to seek: the specificity of the case with AIDS lies in its the close association with homosexuality and drug abuse, and hence with sin. Assuming, as is still more often than not the case in the West, that a person has contracted the virus through one of these two illicit practices, the following problem arises: does Halakhah recognize an obligation to extend help to sufferers whom one assumes to have contracted the illness through a sinful act? Should this person be provided with medical care just like any other patient, or is his or her presumed prior sinful activity, which in the first place *caused the illness*, relevant in one way or another? The issue has been very pointedly formulated by Dr. Fred Rosner:

> The Sabbath must be desecrated to save a human life. But is the desecration of the Sabbath allowed and/or mandated to save the life of a sinner who is guilty of a crime such as homosexuality for which the death penalty might be imposed?[62]

The (felicitous) fact of the matter is that on this issue a wide, clear, and unequivocal consensus prevails—all writers on the matter, including all Orthodox writers, unambiguously uphold that one's obligations toward the sick are invariant with respect to their moral record. Now no less interesting than this reassuring conclusion itself are the various argumentative strategies deployed to sustain it. We will first look at the obligations of the Jewish physician, and then consider the question whether the lay Jew's general obligation to assist the sick applies differently to PWHIVs and PWAs.

To make the point that the physician is obligated to extend help to PWHIVs and PWAs, Rabbi Freundel adduces a particularly forceful argument, which follows the same type of hermeneutic of the Scriptures that underlies his argument that AIDS is likely to be a divine visitation. After Korah and his band are swallowed up by the earth, the Israelites rebel against Moses and Aaron, whereupon God sends a plague to destroy them. Notwithstanding the fact that this plague is explicitly affirmed to be a divine retribution, Moses charges Aaron to carry a firepan with incense from the altar into the midst of the people. By doing this, Aaron indeed brings the plague to a halt.[63] Noting that this Biblical story "parallels the most extreme view of the AIDS situation"—i.e., the view that it is a divine punishment— Freundel concludes:

> The authentic Jewish response consisted of trying to save as many people as possible. The same response should apply in the AIDS crisis, regardless of its origin. . . . It makes no practical difference if AIDS is divine in origin or not. . . . If I am confronted with dangerously ill AIDS patients, my only agenda, as was Aaron's, is to heal them as quickly as possible. *Lo ta'amod al dam re'ekha*—"Do not stand idly on the blood of your neighbor" (Levit. 19:16).[64]

Rabbi Freundel's position is remarkable in that it severs all relationship between the theological interpretation of AIDS and Halakhah. Even if one adopts what Freundel calls "the most extreme view of the AIDS situation," i.e., the view that AIDS is a divine retribution directed against the individual sinner, one is still obligated to treat the PWHIVs and PWAs just like any other patient. Theology and Halakhah are two autonomous, mutually independent realms; the Jew's concrete social obligations as halakhically determined are invariant with respect to his or her theological beliefs.

Professor David Novak reaches the same conclusion, but through a very different line of reasoning. As we saw, he holds, contrary to most other halakhic writers, that PWHIVs and PWAs are mostly "in the category of sinners." Still, he clearly states that this fact "should in no wise prevent full care being extended" to them. Moreover, it is even our obligation to sympathize with them, because according to Jewish tradition everyone is essentially a sinner, so that the "difference between the righteous and the wicked is ultimately one of degree, not of kind."[65] Further, according to the Talmud, one of the reasons why *zara'at* sufferers were put in quarantine was to give them the opportunity to publicly express their pain and "to beseech others to 'seek compassion [*rahamim*] for them.'"[66] Therefore, with regard to these sufferers the community has both a spiritual and a moral involvement.

Dr. Fred Rosner's approach to the issue is entirely different still. According to Halakhah, he argues, all commandments (except idolatry, incest, and murder) are to be waived when this is required to save a human life (*piqquah nefesh*). But does this apply also to sinners, specifically those whose sins entail a death punishment? Rosner's answer is positive. The Talmud, he reports, states that "every life is worth saving without distinction as to whether the person whose life is in danger is a criminal or transgressor or law-abiding citizen."[67] Indeed, according to Halakhah, the Jew's obligation to extend help to a person in danger ceases only when that person is considered "halakhically dead," namely, when he or she is either a *rodef* (i.e., threatening someone else's life) or has been sentenced to death by a Sanhedrin.[68] Since PWHIVs and PWAs, including sinners, fall into neither of these two categories,[69] there is, juridically, no difference between them and anyone else. As a result, although the patient is known to be a transgressor, the physician is obligated to extend help to him or her and even to suspend the commandments in order to save his or her life. Rosner thus states that "it seems clear that patients with AIDS should be treated medically and psychosocially no differently than other patients."[70] Roughly the same position is taken by Dr. Abraham Steinberg.[71]

A very general consideration adduced by Rabbi J. David Bleich complements and reinforces this conclusion. Bleich notes that for over two millennia, punishments for transgressions of the kind of homosexual conduct are no longer imposed, and that the renewed application of the Biblical punishments presupposes the restoration of the Sanhedrin in the Temple. He opines that in the absence of a juridically qualified body to decide in matters of guilt, the entire question of punishment does not at all arise in one's relationship to a transgressor (of whatever commandment). His practical conclusion is the following: "Insofar as our attitude is concerned, the [homosexual] act must be deplored, but the person who commits such acts remains a Jew to whom our hearts and arms are open."[72]

All halakhic authors on the subject, then, including those who tend to view AIDS as a divine retribution (Freundel, Novak) and those for whom homosexuals not only sin but are sinners (Novak), unequivocally state that PWAs and PWHIVs should receive all possible medical and socio-psychological help. That their condition may have its origin in a sinful act is entirely irrelevant to the question of the practical attitude toward them *qua* sufferers.[73] This unanimity is noteworthy and is not to be regarded as a matter of course. The fact that each of our authors grounds his attitude in a different reasoning seems to suggest that taken individually, the arguments are not entirely watertight, with the implication that the issue is halakhically indeterminate, i.e., that a case could be made also for the opposite stance; we will shortly see that this is indeed precisely the case. The consensus among our authors seems to indicate that the opposite stance—advocating that PWHIVs and PWAs should be treated differently than other, more "innocent" patients—is simply not an acceptable option within Judaism.

The historical roots of this attitude are perhaps to be gleaned from a consideration adduced by Dr. Benjamin Freedman:

> Within Judaism, duties toward the ill are, paradoxically, not affected by the reason behind the illness, precisely because the connection between sin and illness is so strong. The traditional belief, rooted in the Bible, was that illness is both caused and sustained by sin: "R. Alexandrai said that R. Chiya bar Aba said, 'The sick one does not stand apart from his sickness until all his sins are forgiven him.'" Inasmuch as there exists this general presumption that illness is caused by sin, were there no duty to care for the *sinful* ill, the duty to care for the ill would never in fact obtain![74]

Healing by physicians was indeed considered illicit by some Jewish authorities, because of the notion that all illness is a punishment from God (this stance is associated, for example, with the name of Nahmanides); despite this tendency, however, an overwhelming and unchallenged consensus seems to have prevailed over the opposite position.[75] This consensus has become an institutionalized norm in Judaism, so much so, indeed, that it cannot be suspended even when (as in the case of AIDS) the etiology involves sinful conduct. Indeed, the consensus about the obligation to succor the ill, and the resulting normative compassion for persons with AIDS, is so dominant that it prevails over other, more legal, considerations pointing in the opposite direction. This thesis can be substantiated by taking cognizance of the fact that the humane attitude is bought at the price of explicit or silent overruling of the Halakhah, a price which those who discuss the problem do not hesitate to pay, be it implicitly, in a concealed manner, or explicitly and openly.

The problem was pointed out by Professor David Novak. Many gays engage in homosexual sex as a way of life and not occasionally. Novak points out that from a halakhic point of view this would seem to mean that they fall into the category of "provocative sinners" (*mumar le-hakh'is*), i.e., people who sin habitually and willfully. Now the Talmud explicitly rules that such sinners must not be helped, and one is even not to save their lives.[76] According to Novak, the only escape from this gruesome conclusion is to declare that strict homosexuals are acting provocatively due to an unnatural inclination, i.e., an illness, so that they can be viewed as acting "under the influence of an unavoidable compulsion (*ones*)."[77] As already noted, however, halakhic authors mostly refuse this move (with the notable exception of Norman Lamm), because it threatens to lead to homosexuality's being recognized as an alternative, gay, way of life that is acceptable within Judaism.[78] In addition, it would lead to the fairly absurd consequence that an occasional homosexual act would be regarded as a transgression deserving capital punishment, whereas homosexuality as a way of life would be regarded as an *ones* and, as such, would not be considered sinful.[79] Strictly, therefore, on the majority's view of homosexuality, Halakhah definitely implies that homosexual PWHIVs and PWAs, especially those who openly declare themselves gay, are "provocative sinners," and, as such, should not be helped. No halakhic thinker, however, is willing to go this far. Consider how they obviate this move.

David Novak poses the problem very clearly: "according to traditional criteria, active homosexuals are provocative sinners." How, then, can one avoid the conclusion that they must not be helped? Novak blatantly states that the Talmudic rulings referring to provocative sinners have been pronounced mainly for educational purposes and must not be taken too literally. Therefore, "this category is subject to a high degree of judicial discretion." Indeed, in the Middle Ages, too, sanctions were applied only to persons who endangered the community. Novak also appeals to the authority of the Hazon Ish, who, as already mentioned, emphasized that the application of halakhic rules to concrete situations should always be subject to an appreciation of what is opportune in a given time and place.[80] Novak thus explicitly recognizes the need to "inactivate," as it were, a Talmudic rule in order to allow for help to be extended to PWHIVs and PWAs who are "provocative sinners."

The avenues open to Novak are not all open to writers defining themselves as Orthodox. Thus, Dr. Fred Rosner, responding to Novak's argument and perhaps feeling uncomfortable with explicit statements concerning the need for "judicial discretion," seeks to avoid saying in so many words that the Talmudic ruling on provocative sinners must not be applied. His way out of the difficulty, it must, however, be said, consists in sweeping the problem under the rug. Whereas provocative sinners are those who sin habitually and willfully, he writes, "one who only occasionally sins out of lust or appetite is considered like one whose life and property are to be protected and carefully treated." And despite the fact that many, perhaps most, homosexuals are gays who obviously cannot be assigned to this category, he proceeds: "It would seem *therefore* that physicians and other health personnel have an obligation to care for patients with AIDS no differently than for other patients";[81] the difficult problem concerning declared gays, i.e., of willful sinners, is not mentioned again. Dr. Abraham Steinberg similarly obfuscates the issue.[82] Other writers, e.g., Bleich and Jakobovits, do not take any notice of the distinction between occasional and provocative sinners. By contrast, the Israeli ultra-Orthodox Rav Yoseph Shalom Elyashiv seems to hold that the cases of those who practice homosexuality occasionally and of those who are homosexuals *lehakh'is* are indeed not on a par.[83]

The preceding consideration shows, I believe, that in order to be able to maintain that medical assistance must be extended to all HIV and AIDS sufferers regardless of their possible status as provocative sinners, one *must* exert, either explicitly or implicitly, "judicial discretion." This seems to substantiate the claim made above according to which the halakhic reasoning on issues related to AIDS is implicitly subjected to an overriding, primary value, that of assisting the sick.[84] Contrary to the theological questions, which are matters of debate, the practical issue of helping PWHIVs and PWAs is the subject of a universal consensus, because the societal norms institutionalized in Judaism apparently make an attitude of rejection into an unacceptable option. Furthermore, it should be realized that taking a different stance on the issue would have resulted in a strictly absurd and untenable position: persons known as provocative sinners because of continual transgressions other than homosexuality— e.g., those who regularly and publicly desecrate the Sabbath or who eat unkosher food—are, of course, not excluded from medical care by any Jewish thinker or decisor: why, then, should homosexuality be the only transgression to justify such a sanction? Indeed, the very fact that homosexuality is the sole sin with respect to which the issue is even raised allows us to recognize, I think, that behind Novak's very throwing up of the problematic concerning the legitimacy of succoring provocative homosexual sinners looms his view of AIDS as a divine punishment. Only if one views AIDS as a divine retribution for homosexuality is it meaningful to single out homosexuality as a sin which, alone among all provocative sins, disqualifies those committing it from receiving medical aid, since the aim of that aid is to alleviate precisely the malady contracted through the sin.

Let me now emphasize the following point: the problematic of homosexual activity is not purely juridical; rather, as can easily be perceived in the writings on the subject, the rejection of homosexuality, for all its juridic foundation, is also strongly charged on the affective level: most of the authors do not conceal that homosexuality is highly repugnant to them. It is therefore significant, and indeed commendable, that none of these authors has let his personal revulsion influence his considered attitude. In fact, social traditionalism (including the rejection of homosexuality) and the belief that God punishes deviation from traditional norms have been found to be factors in the rejection of AIDS sufferers.[85] Even certain health care providers, not necessarily Jewish, let their homophobia negatively influence their attitude toward AIDS patients.[86] Similarly, certain Christian officials have expressed reluctance to extend help to PWA, lest this action be interpreted as condoning the (presumed) cause of AIDS, namely, homosexuality.[87] It would seem again that the general Jewish value of the importance of assisting suffering persons was a decisive factor in determining the positions. In the American setting, especially, in which quite vociferous spokesmen for Christian fundamentalism and others have taken the opposite stand—"even the traditionally sacrosanct public commitment to the medical treatment of the sick was not spared the assault of those who viewed AIDS as emblematic of the moral degradation of society," as one author commented[88]—this should be particularly appreciated.[89] In sum, then, it is perhaps not simplistic and naive to say that the imperative of helping the sick is a supreme value in Judaism that, despite a strong traditional homophobia and irrespective of all specific halakhic considerations, rules out an attitude of rejection toward suffering persons.[90] In fact, statements and resolutions by Jewish religious and secular bodies have in common that they all carry a paragraph strongly urging that the ill be succored—namely, to perform the commandment of *biqqur holim* (to which we will return back below).

* * *

A question related to the one just discussed is whether and to what extent health personnel are obligated to expose themselves to a health risk in order to extend assistance to PWHIVs and PWAs. From a halakhic perspective, the question largely hinges on the degree of danger involved in contacts with PWHIVs and PWAs. Dr. Fred Rosner briefly reviews the history of rulings on the issue of whether and to what extent one should undergo a risk in order to succor someone else (there are two distinct and coexisting traditions, going back to the two Talmuds) and concludes that the prevailing opinion among rabbinic decisors is as follows:

> If there is great danger to the rescuer, he is not allowed to attempt to save his fellow man; if he nevertheless does so, he is called a pious fool; if the danger to the rescuer is small and the danger to his fellow man very great, the rescuer is allowed but not obligated to attempt the rescue, and if he does so his act is called an act of loving-kindness (*midat hasidut*). If there is no risk at all to the rescuer or if the risk is very small or remote, he is obligated to try to save his fellow man. If he refuses to do so, he is guilty of transgressing the commandment *thou shalt not stand idly by the blood of thy fellow man* (Lev. 19:16).[91]

Dr. Rosner concludes from this consensual ruling that "since the risk to physicians and other health personnel in caring for AIDS patients is infinitesimally small (less than a fraction of 1 percent), it follows that a physician is obligated under Jewish law to care for such patients."[92] This is also the opinion of other authors who have addressed the question.[93]

An especially interesting approach to the question has been put forward by Professor David Novak. He deduces the physician's obligation to heal not from Maimonides's account (which grounds the obligation of restoring health on that of restoring lost property), but rather from the approach of Nahmanides. The latter construes the physician's activity as an *imitatio Dei*, analogous to the activity of a judge, and derives from this the idea that the physician is obligated to heal, just as the judge is obligated to judge. Novak points out that this construal has a decisive advantage over the Maimonidean approach: since AIDS is not a curable illness, anchoring the physician's obligation to heal in Maimonides' notion of the obligation to *restore* health falls to the ground. By contrast, viewing healing as a divine commandment anchored in the example of divine activity upholds and buttresses the notion that "Judaism obligates care."[94]

It is another question whether a lay person is required to extend help to PWHIVs and PWAs. From a halakhic point of view, this question is theoretically different from the preceding one because there is no "rescuing" involved here. Nonetheless, since no danger at all results from casual contact with PWAs,[95] visiting those suffering from AIDS is clearly obligatory.[96] Indeed, the commandment to visit the sick—*biqqur holim*—is highly underscored not only by all individual writers on AIDS, but also by the official bodies of all denominations of Judaism.[97] The reason for this is that, although as a point of *fact* casual contact with PWHIVs and PWAs involves no danger whatsoever, AIDS is still perceived as a menacing disease; the insistence on the mitzvah of *biqqur holim* is thus addressed to those who fear that such a contact may put them in danger.[98]

Questions of Prevention

We may now consider some further practical problems raised by halakhic authors and try to relate the answers they suggest to their value-systems and their theological and halakhic commitments.

First and foremost among these practical questions is that concerning prevention. The preventive measures taken by state sanitary authorities the world over consist, as is well known, in advocating the use of condoms, to prevent the transmission of HIV during sexual contact, and in facilitating the access of intravenous drug users to clean needles, to prevent contagion through the shared use of needles. Now from a halakhic point of view, both of these measures are highly problematic, because they apply essentially to illegal situations. Extramarital sex and, *a fortiori*, homosexual sex are forbidden, and indeed, even the use of a condom by a married couple, although under discussion, is prohibited by most authorities in the great majority of situations;[99] the very use of drugs, too, is proscribed by Halakhah. The practical efficiency of these preventive strategies therefore confronts the halakhic Jewish thinker with the following dilemma: joining the secular authorities in advocating these preventive measures amounts to recognizing—*de facto*, although not *de jure*—the existence, indeed the prevalence, of forbidden practices and forms of life among Jews; alternatively, by abstaining from joining the educative campaigns in favor of these measures, one takes the risk of passively contributing to the spread of a lethal illness. Orthodox Jewish thinkers, we will now see, are almost unanimous in refusing to endorse preventive measures running against the Halakhah.

Rabbi Jakobovits is, once again, particularly clear: "I cannot accept anything which publicly condones or encourages immorality. The present campaign does. By speaking of 'safe sex' or 'safer sex', and by advising on recourse to condoms . . . the campaign officially accepts some form of extra-marital relations as the norm. . . . Altogether, in effect the campaign encourages promiscuity by advertising it. It tells people not what is right, but how to do wrong and get away with it."[100] For Rabbi Jakobovits, then, the campaign in favor of the use of condoms is ill-advised, and he urges, instead, "the cultivation of new attitudes calculated to restore reverence for the generation of life and the enjoyment of sexual pleasures exclusively within marriage."[101] He calls, not for piecemeal pragmatical steps which sanction the evil instead of eradicating it, but rather for a total social transformation of attitudes toward sex and family: "Nothing short of a moral revolution will in time contain the scourge."[102] Lord Jakobovits calls for a moral revolution that will once again make the Jewish people a "light for the Nations"; just as Abraham prayed for Sodom, in which there was not a single Jew, so the Jews of today are obligated to rescue the sinful generation by diffusing the message that "more important than clean needles are clean thoughts and clean conduct."[103]

Can it not be argued that the absolute primacy the Jewish tradition accords to the saving of life sanctions both the use of condoms (even by unmarried persons) and the distribution of clean needles? This position has been advocated, for instance, by René-Samuel Sirat, former Chief Rabbi of France and current President of the Permanent Council of the Conference of European Rabbis. After proclaiming that the true answer to AIDS is fidelity within the married couple—"we should give moral guidance and not say 'use condoms to avert the illness'"—Rabbi Sirat added:

> But it is also our duty to say to those whom we address that the greatest crime would be to heap upon lewdness also the danger of contaminating one or more partners. It is of primary importance to underscore that those who are incapable of controlling their sexual lusts, and who may therefore infect those with whom they share intimacy, should be mindful to protect their own life as well as that of their eventual partners.[104]

As could be expected, this moderate position is upheld by rabbis of the less strict Jewish denominations. Thus Rabbi W. Gunther Plaut of the CCAR writes with complete clarity:

> Life is precious and must be saved under all circumstances and at all costs. While ordinarily the ends do not sanctify the means and the religious law must not be infringed for otherwise desirable purposes, it is different when it comes to the preservation of life and, by implication, the prevention of pandemic disease.
> Prevention of HIV transmission may involve providing means for sexual activity which in itself is frowned upon by much of Jewish tradition. The liberal view (taken by the presenter) holds that the preservation of life must be paramount, and that all possible support must be given to programs which will prevent people from becoming infected and from infecting others.[105]

Rabbi Jakobovits had anticipated—and rejected—Sirat's and Plaut's argument: "even this pro-life stance [within Judaism] has three cardinal exceptions: forbidden liaisons, murder and idolatry are proscribed even at the cost of life. This, too, would seem to rule out recourse to any measures, such as condoms for unmarrieds, which would encourage indecent conduct, though the rule might be invoked to treat more leniently the distribution of clean needles for drug-abusers."[106] Jakobovits finds support for his position in the decision of the fifteenth-century Spanish-Jewish scholar Isaac Arama, who objected to the establishment of communally-controlled brothels as a means of lessening the capital offense of adultery.[107] His argument was that the pragmatical benefits of mitigating individual sinful activity cannot be bought at the expense of "the slightest public compromise with the Divine Law."[108] Similarly, Dr. Abraham Steinberg writes:

> The directives for "safe sex" as given today, which are in fact directives for homosexual sex, are incompatible with the Torah. Nor can one assent to the directives to distribute sterile needles to drug-addicts; rather, the addiction should be fought against. From a Jewish point of view, there is no difference between the two battles. An educational campaign should therefore emphasize the negative aspects in the behavior of the risk-groups—homosexuals, drug-addicts, and prostitutes. . . . Since there is a chance for education against sexual deviance to be effective, more efforts should be made in this direction.[109]

Other Orthodox rabbis do not even raise the issue of the use of condoms by unmarrieds: it is simply beyond their horizon. Orthodox authors, we see, for the most part refuse "to legislate within illegal situations," to use Rabbi Rivon Krygier's felicitous phrase.[110] It would seem that they fear that taking cognizance of the existence of the societal reality of illegal situations could amount to—or be interpreted as—recognizing them as legitimate. Rather than enter upon what they feel is a slippery slope, they prefer to limit their message to the binary one of an "all or nothing" logic. They address themselves to their own—Orthodox—community, whose norms indeed make the use of condoms unnecessary; and as for the rest of Jewish society, either it engages in a total change of morals—i.e., in a moral *revolution*—or else Orthodox Judaism has no message for it. Rabbi Jakobovits's use of the term "revolution"—"Only a Moral Revolution Can Contain This Scourge" was the title of his December 1986 *Times* article[111]—is indeed significant. Just as Marxist revolutionaries refused to engage in possibly progressive piecemeal improvements of society—i.e., in social reform or better perhaps, *social technology* as advocated by the late Sir Karl R. Popper—arguing that only the total replacement of the existing social order by an alternative one could remedy social evils, so too Orthodox thinkers (with the notable exception of Rabbi Sirat) reject merely practical measures aimed at reducing the spread of HIV in the currently existing society, and urge a total upheaval of social, specifically sexual mores.

The Balance of Individual Rights and Public Good in Halakhah: Screening and Confidentiality

We now come to issues bearing on the balance of two often-conflicting values and rights, namely, the public good, and more specifically the public health, on the one hand, and personal freedom and autonomy, on the other. The problem, as one author has felicitously put it, is to strike a balance "that protects those who have the disease and which also protects the healthy from the disease."[112] Public health policy in matters of epidemics has traditionally been based on coercive, compulsory, and restrictive measures, usually directed specifically against pre-sumed high-risk groups that more often than not were also socially marginal. The fact that these measures were at variance with the principles of individual liberty and unrestricted auton-omy was hardly noticed during earlier pandemics, even in the early twentieth century; an awareness of the conflict between the rights of the individual and the considerations guiding pub-lic heath has arisen only with appearance of AIDS.[113] In fact, in every country the balance between these two conflicting inter-ests is continuously struck anew as a result of ongoing political struggles.[114]

Social philosophers all have their own stances on whether and how these two sets of values and principles can be harmo-nized, either theoretically or pragmatically. Our objective in what follows will be to see how Jewish thinkers endeavor to elaborate answers to this quandary that are grounded in the Halakhah. Two issues are at the center of the debate over public health vs. individual rights: mandatory screening, and the right to confidentiality of medical information. We will consider them in turn.

1. Let us take screening up first. Owing to principled concerns about personal freedom and also to the more pragmatic fear that mandatory testing could drive persons at risk away from treat-ment and thereby negatively interfere with prevention strate-

gies, universal mandatory screening has been rejected in all but one country, except in certain specific contexts, such as prisons, the army, or hospitals.[115] The positions of Orthodox Jewish writers would seem to fall to the right of this universal consensus.

Rabbi J. David Bleich believes that the Jewish position is clearly in favor of mandatory screening programs, if these give the promise of contributing to diminishing the spread of AIDS. His argument follows two complementary lines. He urges, first, that personal autonomy is not a Jewish value, and second, that the collective good is. In Bleich's view, individual rights are not anchored in Jewish law. Rather, if a specific individual right is to be recognized as such by Judaism, it must be promulgated by an appropriate rabbinical ordinance. A case in point is Rabbenu Gershom's interdiction on reading one's neighbor's mail. The right to privacy, Bleich reasons, is not inherent in, and therefore cannot be derived from, Jewish law, whence the need to legislate separately on every aspect of it. Thus, in Jewish law there is no "right" of the individual ruling out mandatory screening programs. On the contrary: according to Bleich, Jewish law in fact supports such testing, indeed justifies making it mandatory. "Judaism," he writes, "posited something akin to the notion of compelling state interest long before that concept arose in American constitutional law. In the case of an individual who poses a threat to society, the individual's rights to autonomy and integrity of his person are subordinated to the needs of society to the extent necessary to eliminate the perceived threat."[116] The halakhic justification for this stance is found in the notion of the *rodef* (pursuer): if an individual threatens the life of another, innocent, person, the pursuer's life can be taken if this is necessary to eliminate the danger; nay, his or her life *must* be taken, should doing so be required to preserve the life of the potential victim. Bleich emphasizes two salient points in this context: First, the pursuer him- or herself may be entirely innocent; his or her being classified as a *rodef*, with the consequence that his or her life is no longer under the protection of the law, is solely the outcome of objective circumstances that make one into a danger to someone else.[117] Second, the obligation to kill the pursuer is binding not only for the potential victim, but also for any third party; consequently, society too is not only authorized to take any action that can save a threatened innocent life, but is even mandated to do so. According to Bleich, then, the notion of *rodef* warrants the following general conclusion: "Judaism clearly recognizes that society has the right to interfere with the exercise of individual autonomy and to infringe upon the liberty of its members in order to protect the lives of members of society at large."[118] The answer to the question whether or not testing for AIDS should be made compulsory therefore hinges on a *factual* question: if it is shown that, in point of fact, such tests give the promise of saving lives, then society not only has the right to institute them, but is under the clear obligation to do so.[119] In sum, "The concerns that augur in favor of mandatory testing programs for identification of the AIDS carriers are certainly quite compelling. . . . The crucial problem is practical rather than theoretical; the most significant problem is how to design and implement testing programs that will effectively protect the lives and health of members of society at large."[120]

That the importance accorded to the autonomy of the individual in the traditional Jewish framework is of a subordinate rank in comparison with other values is emphasized in this context by Dr. Abraham Steinberg. All the laws in a civil society, to one degree or another, restrict individual freedom, he argues, and Judaism advocates such restrictions even more forcefully:

> According to Judaism, any religious and moral obligation nullifies the autonomy of the individual. Therefore one cannot draw on the principles of individual freedom or self-determination to sanction whatever transgression, even if it involves no harm to a third party. In other words: not only stealing and murder cannot be justified through the claim of autonomy, but the same holds also of violating the Sabbath, eating pork, etc. According to Judaism, [individual] autonomy is restricted to such kinds of behavior that involve no damage or harm—neither to oneself nor to someone else—where "harm" is defined according to the commands of the Torah.[121]

Two corollaries follow. For one thing, from a Jewish point of view, the principle of autonomy must not be used to condone homosexuality.[122] Second, and more directly relevant in the present context, in Judaism the principle of autonomy is only one among many principles, and it can be allowed to guide one's action only when not contradicted by another, higher principle.[123] Now as the considerations based on the notion of *rodef* show, Halakhah gives precedence to the principle of preserving the well-being of potential victims and, by implication, of the entire public, over the principle of autonomy. Consequently, Halakhah authorizes and even makes it obligatory for the public to take measures to protect itself, specifically to institute mandatory screening, should it prove to be an efficient means of preventing the spread of the pandemic.

The same position is defended, although on the basis of a somewhat different argument, by Rav Shlomo Deichowsky, a member of the Rabbinical Court of Appeals in Israel. Mandatory screening is warranted, he asserts, for the good both of those tested and of society at large. He construes the high-risk groups—especially homosexuals and intravenous drug users—as being in the halakhic situation of a plague. According to various rulings, during a plague, all measures, including even those that involve violations of important religious precepts, are permitted in order to save lives. For instance, it is not only allowed, but even imperative, to eat on Yom Kippur, when this can be expected to strengthen the body's resistance to the threat of a plague. Consequently, since the high-risk groups are to be viewed as living within a plague, compulsory measures which follow the aim of saving lives, including screening, are warranted and even mandatory.[124]

The public good, too, sanctions such measures. Like Bleich, Deichowsky grounds this position on the notion of *rodef*: "It is known that high-risk groups endanger not only their own members, but also the general population. Therefore, even if they so endanger the general population without evil intent, their members are subsumable under the law of the pursuer. It should be noted that the law of the pursuer applies even in cases of doubt [*safeq rodef*]."[125] Lastly, lest these halakhic demonstrations should be thought inconclusive, Deichowsky also invokes the rule of *migdar milta*, i.e., the power of the city elders to temporally enact whatever extraordinary rules or sanctions they see fit, including such that have no foundation in the Torah, if they deem them necessary to check a risk or a danger.[126] "And surely no measure aiming to check a danger is of greater importance than one intended to prevent the contamination of many people by a deadly, incurable illness," Deichowsky writes, "when all that is required of the members of the high-risk group is a simple blood test."[127]

Rav Deichowsky's reasoning is faulty on more than one count, it would seem to me. His argument in favor of screening, which is grounded in the good of the persons to be tested, obviously proceeds on the premise that violating the integrity of an individual's body is legitimate in the interest of his or her own health. Deichowsky ignores the conspicuous fact that no cure to AIDS is available today, so that the proposed measures *do not* give the promise of saving the lives of seropositives or AIDS patients.[128] Consequently, the precedents invoked by Deichowsky—e.g., eating on Yom Kippur to thwart the danger to one's life—are simply not relevant; until such time as a cure for AIDS is found, the situations are *not analogous*. Moreover, to buttress his argument that mandatory testing is warranted because it is carried out (also) for the benefit of the members of the risk-group themselves, R. Deichowsky writes (perhaps anticipating the above objection): "Although the disease is as yet incurable, there is no doubt that timely intervention may lengthen the patient's life."[129] But this argument may also be fallacious, for it proceeds on a factual premise which is not necessarily true, inasmuch as at present (mid- 1996), early treatment *does not* prolong life, nor does it even improve its quality.[130]

Rav Deichowsky's argument grounded in the public good is also fallacious. It hinges on the premise that the high-risk groups are to be construed as a *rodef* (or *safeq rodef*) of the general population, which is problematical for at least two reasons. First, it applies to a *group* a notion that has usually been applied only to individuals, an extension whose validity is questionable because not everyone in the *rodef* group is necessarily a *rodef*. Second, and more important, the notion of *rodef* presupposes an entirely passive and innocent victim (the paradigmatic case is that of a rape), a situation that hardly ever applies to the present case, where the virus is typically transmitted in situations involving two *consenting* actors, whose relevant action (extramarital or homosexual sex or drug abuse), moreover, is sinful from the point of view of Jewish law.[131]

Rabbi Jakobovits refuses to take a stand on the issue of mandatory testing, and it is noteworthy that, contrary to Bleich, he does not draw on the notion of *rodef* to analyze it. He contents himself with avowing his perplexity, which is humane and pragmatic rather than strictly halakhic: "Other problems, too, are baffling and defy any definitive answers: for instance, whether, as widely advocated, we should increasingly think of compulsory testing of people to discover if they are carriers or not. . . . To whom would one communicate the result—the patient on whom one would thereby inflict a shattering trauma, or others who would then ostracize the patient or otherwise discriminate against him? All these are frightful questions for which no immediate and reliable answers can yet be found."[132]

2. A related issue is that of confidentiality. Should a positive result, whether obtained through individual testing or through screening, be made available only to the infected person, or to others (relatives, medical workers, etc.) as well? Secular thought on the issue is again oriented by two considerations: the pragmatic one relating to public health, and the principled one relating to the individual's right to privacy. We will now see that Halakhah is indeterminate on the issue and that Orthodox writers hold conflicting views of it.

Rabbi J. David Bleich's extensive discussion of this issue proceeds in two steps. Bleich first establishes that the two possible positions on the issue can both claim to have a foundation in Jewish law. On the one hand, Jewish law establishes the general principle of confidentiality by virtue of the interdiction of *lashon ha-ra'*. The commandment "You shall not go as a bearer of tales among your people" (Lev. 19:16) "prohibits gossip-mongering even if the information divulged in no way results in substantive harm or prejudice to the interests of the person whose affairs are divulged," R. Bleich writes; gossip (even innocent gossip) is a "serious transgression of divine law."[133] Generally speaking, therefore, Judaism warrants confidentiality in matters medical.

This consideration is also deemed to be overriding to two eminent ultra-Orthodox Israeli rabbinic authorities, Rav Yoseph Shalom Elyashiv and his son-in-law Rav Yitzhaq Zilberstein. They disallowed the publication of the name of an AIDS patient even though he was known to intentionally and willingly spread the illness as an act of vengeance. They grounded their decision mainly on two arguments: first, the doors of repentance (teshuvah) should not be shut, and as long as the sinner's shame (i.e., presumably his homosexuality) has not become generally known, he may yet repent, whereas if its knowledge has spread, he will despair and not repent; second, by publicizing the name of the patient, his family is harmed too, and this must be prevented in accordance with the prohibition of gossip-mongering. Indeed, they ruled that even after the death of an AIDS patient it is forbidden to make public the nature of his or her illness, so as not to embarrass the family.[134] To them, then, the imperative of protecting privacy prevails over all other considerations.

Rabbi Bleich, however, follows a different line of reasoning. In his view, the interdiction of talebearing is not the only general principle of Jewish law relevant to the analysis of the question of confidentiality. This is because, if privacy is protected under all circumstances, then some PWHIVs and PWAs may behave irresponsibly and spread the disease. Not informing third parties (sexual partners, medical workers, etc.) may thus imply putting their lives in danger. Contrary to the ruling of Rav Elyashiv and Rav Zilberstein (of which he was unaware), he holds that this is prohibited by Jewish law.[135]

In Rabbi Bleich's view, then, two distinct halakhic principles with contradictory implications are relevant to the question of confidentiality. Where two Jewish values are in conflict, Bleich argues, we should examine their relative places in "the hierarchical ranking of values that is reflected through . . . Jewish law."[136] In the present case, the outcome of this examination is quite clear: "under such circumstances [in which a seropositive person is assumed to behave irresponsibly], protection of human life should take precedence over preservation of professional secrecy."[137] Thus, as a matter of principle, confidentiality is not an absolute value, and it must be violated where doing so gives the promise of saving lives.

So much for the principled considerations. But reality is here more complex than neat principles, as R. Bleich recognizes in the wake of debates among secular authors on medical ethics. The problem is whether adopting a policy that permits divulging a given person's serological status to third parties may not, in the long run and as a point of empirical fact, result in having effects that are just the opposite of what was intended. The argument is this: Contravening confidentiality is done with the thought that conferring absolute value upon confidentiality would put innocent lives in danger. Yet it is possible that if this policy becomes known, people, especially those who are at risk, may be slow to come forward for testing, for fear that their positive serological status may eventually become known to third parties. If this is indeed so, then obviously breaking confidentiality may increase, rather than diminish, the number of deaths.

So far the "genuine moral dilemma,"[138] which confronts secular thinkers on medical ethics and health politicians in exactly the same terms. Common sense would suggest that the principled solution depends on factual information; we should adopt the policy that gives the promise of saving the greatest number of lives. This is also Rabbi Bleich's position, although he correctly notes that the empirical information at our disposal is insufficient to decide the issue.[139] Yet to sustain this principled stance, Bleich first has to make a halakhic point. The reason is this: those whose lives will be saved if confidentiality is broken are identifiable individuals, namely, persons in contact with specific PWHIVs and PWAs; by contrast, those whose lives will be saved if a policy of strict confidentiality is adopted "exist only as a statistical probability."[140] In other words: the "ontic status" (if this expression be allowed) of the two kinds of persons whose lives are to be saved is not the same, and comparing the two groups numerically is therefore problematic. A halakhic discussion of the notion of danger is thus necessary to decide whether or not the saving of unidentified potential victims outweighs the saving of identifiable victims, warranting the eventual overruling of the imperative of confidentiality.

Rabbi Bleich's analysis of the issue is as follows: It is well known that precepts may be violated for the benefit of an ill person. As a rule, this refers to a concrete, identified individual (the situation of *holeh lefanenu*). Yet, according to Rabbinic authorities (notably the Hazon Ish, Rabbi Isser Yehudah Unterman), the existence of an *identifiable danger* (e.g., a plague) threatening a group puts all members of that group into the category of "identifiable ill persons" for whose sake commandments may be violated. This means that in order for such a violation to be warranted, it is enough that the *danger* be identifiable; any member of the menaced group is then sufficiently identified as to warrant construing him as a *holeh lefanenu*. Thus the general conclusion is that the "statistical probability of danger constitutes the halakhic equivalent of *holeh lefanenu*,"[141] and so, generally, "statistically predictable events are [to be] treated as present dangers."[142] Rabbi Bleich confirms this halakhic reasoning by two examples appealing to the sense of natural justice.[143]

Thus the upshot of the discussion is that there is no principled difference between, on the one hand, the identifiable persons who are at risk through their contact with a given PWHIV or PWA and who can be saved by breaking confidentiality, and, on the other hand, the unidentifiable persons "out there" who will be put at risk through a general policy of breaking confidentiality. It thus follows, just as on secular ethical considerations, that our final decision will depend on a point of actual *fact*: "If it were to be established that identification of AIDS victims and divulgence of that information to sexual partners would ultimately result in the loss of a greater number of lives, a case could well be made for passively refraining from disclosing that information."[144]

Under certain conditions, then, which have to do with *realia*, namely, with the repercussions of the breach of confidentiality on the behaviors of persons at risk, Halakhah thus unambiguously implies, according to Bleich's own analysis, that, by virtue of the principle of *piqquah nefesh*, confidentiality must be respected. This position would seem to be elegant for three reasons: it entirely subsumes the issue of confidentiality under the value of saving a maximal number of lives; it is in accord with the interdiction of *lashon ha-ra'*; and it aligns Halakhah with "general" medical ethics. It is therefore quite remarkable that Rabbi Bleich does not rest content with this result. Instead, he engages in a long discussion aimed at eating the cake and having it too. Bleich describes a model intended to allow both (mandatory) screening *and* selective informing of partners (i.e., partners of seropositives who do not offer sufficient guarantees that they protect them) without the latter's counterproductive effects.[145] The model itself is of little interest for us here. For our purposes, the significant point seems to be this: whereas Halakhah would allow Rabbi Bleich to adopt what is generally viewed as a "liberal" position on confidentiality—namely, that of protecting the seropositive person's right to privacy, even at the expense of putting third parties in risk—he goes out of his way not to do so; and he does it through an entirely secular process of reasoning and model construction in which Halakhah plays no part whatsoever. This would seem to point to the following conclusion: Bleich adopts his position on confidentiality not because it is entailed by Halakhah with necessity, but, so it would seem, because it suits his generally conservative temper and inclinations. The comparison with the ruling of the Israeli rabbis Elyashiv and Zilberstein, which was grounded solely in considerations relating to *lashon ha-ra'*, would seem to support the interpretation that Rabbi Bleich's considerations (consciously or not) involved extra-halakhic values.

Conclusion

Looking at the issues discussed by Jewish authors in connection with AIDS sheds interesting light not only on specific questions pertaining to the treatment of AIDS in Judaism, but, more broadly, on Judaism itself. By observing how Judaism tackles the new problems raised by AIDS, one finds that AIDS itself can at the same time become instrumental as an analytical tool affording insights into the nature of Judaism. Following this line of thought, I suggest the following observations, some of which have already been made in passing earlier.

The most consequential factor concerning the perception and handling of AIDS in Judaism seems to be the pervasive notion that AIDS is inherently connected with homosexuality. Although it has never been true that all PWHIVs and PWAs contracted their malady through homosexuality or drug abuse,[146] AIDS has still been stereotyped as the "gay disease," and this has deeply affected all discussions of the subject within Judaism. This is manifest not only in the debate over whether AIDS is to be construed as a divine visitation, but also in discussions of more strictly halakhic questions, such as those concerning confidentiality. Thus, most authorities, as we have seen, rule that revealing to third parties the fact that a person is seropositive or has AIDS may embarrass the family even if done after the person's death, and is a transgression of the interdiction on *lashon ha-ra'*. Since similar strict rulings have not been issued with respect, say, to coronary diseases, it is clear that the salient factor is not the affliction as such, but rather its presumed sinful origin; in the minds of the Jewish authors who wrote on AIDS (as with many other writers on the subject), AIDS is still inextricably bound up with homosexuality or drug abuse.

In the light of this shared perception of AIDS as an affliction whose origin is intrinsically connected with sin, it is noteworthy that our authors *do not* share a common theological interpretation of the significance of AIDS, while they *do share* the view that PWHIVs and PWAs fall under the obligation of *biqqur holim* and must be helped.

As has been seen, there is no consistency within Judaism, and not even within Orthodox Judaism, over the *theological* significance of the AIDS pandemic. While some authors are strongly inclined to view AIDS as a divine visitation, others forcefully reject any such suggestion. It is also noteworthy that even those authors who incline toward the view that AIDS is a divine punishment suggest this view prudently rather than affirm it blatantly and unequivocally; the virulent discourse of Christian fundamentalism is altogether absent from Judaism. Jewish thinkers tend to view AIDS as the natural result of man's tempering with the divinely instituted natural-*cum*-moral equilibrium of the universe. They consequently urge that "only a moral revolution can contain this scourge."

We have also seen that all authors, irrespective of their theological construal of AIDS, unanimously hold that it is incumbent upon Jews (both health personnel and lay people) to help the ill. The halakhic consideration that some AIDS sufferers may be provocative sinners and, as such, must *not* be helped is explicitly or implicitly disregarded. It would seem that assisting the suffering is a value so strongly anchored in Judaism that it can be undone neither by any halakhic consideration nor by the traditional Jewish homophobia. At the same time, the writers repeatedly insist that sympathy for the suffering should in no way be interpreted as an expression of sympathy for their (assumed) style of life.

That extra-halakhic considerations and values may intervene in determining an author's response to a given issue has been noted also elsewhere. We have seen that by virtue of the interdiction of *lashon ha-ra'*, the purely halakhic considerations unambiguously warrant the unmitigated imperative of confidentiality. Still, some authors advocate the violating of confidentiality in the interest of third parties, following what in secular discussions is considered to be a broadly conservative, rather than a liberal, approach to the issue. It would seem that in matters of AIDS some positions are taken not because they are strictly implied and necessitated by Halakhah, but because they are consonant with certain extra-halakhic values. These may be Jewish values, as in the case of helping the sick, or secular ones, as in the case of violating confidentiality.

Notes

1. AIDS = Acquired Immunodeficiency Syndrome; HIV = Human Immunodeficiency Virus. HIV is the etiological agent of AIDS.

2. See, however, "Response to AIDS by the Jewish Community in the United States" (below, p. 135–138), for a short account.

3. This is largely recognized today; see Shilts, *And the Band Played On.*

4. Unterman, "Judaism and Homosexuality," p. 7. Unterman spiritedly brings out the absurdity of this stance from a halakhic point of view: "It is rather as if groups were formed within the Orthodox community which defined themselves as 'The Union of Jewish Adulterers,' 'Jewish Lovers of Pork,' or 'Pesach Bread-Eaters'" (ibid.).

5. For a useful overview of Roman Catholic attitudes toward homosexuality, see Zion, "AIDS and Homosexuality."

6. The terms "AIDS patient," "AIDS victim," and their cognates are not welcome today: "*PWA* (person with AIDS). Identity label developed by people who were suffering from complications of AIDS to destigmatize two of the metaphors used to characterize AIDS, the metaphors of death and punishment, which found their way into everyday discourse in terms such as 'AIDS victim,' 'invariably fatal,' 'promiscuous,' 'AIDS patient,' and 'innocent victim.' This redefinition process was a means by which an emphasis could be put on processes of living and dying, with dignity and without blame, and on a person's ability to take control of his or her life. The initials were picked up by others; PWARC and PWHIV were used as abbreviations, respectively, for persons with AIDS-related complex and persons with HIV infection." Huber and Schneider, eds., *The Social Context of AIDS*, p. 182. Cf. also Mann, Tarantola, and Netter, eds., *AIDS in the World*, p. 539n. My adoption of this "identity label" does not signal that I entirely concur with the motivations that underlay its introduction, nor is it motivated by a wish to follow a "politically correct" line. Rather, it is used out of respect for the self-definition and self-perception of PWA and PWHIV themselves.

7. As one author has fittingly put it: "Gay people with AIDS present the church with a dilemma of status in that they are simultaneously 'sick' and 'sinners.'" Kowalewski, *All Things to All People*, p. 1.

8. Lamm, "Judaism and the Modern Attitude to Homosexuality," p. 213. An original, complementary, view was expressed more recently by Rabbi Hillel Goldberg in his "Homosexuality: A Religious and Political Analysis" (see below, n. 78). See also Unterman, "Judaism and Homosexuality."

9. The term "halakhic writers" designates writers who argue within the framework of the Halakhah, rather than from a postulated system of Jewish values.

10. For the views on homosexuality presupposed in discussions of AIDS, see, e.g., Rosner, "The Acquired Immunodeficiency Syndrome (AIDS): Jewish Perspectives," pp. 177–178; Bleich, "AIDS: A Jewish Perspective," pp. 51–52; Jakobovits, "Halachic Perspectives on AIDS," below, p. 15; Novak, "The Problem of AIDS," below, pp. 81–82. One author who embraces Lamm's position and brings it to bear on the issue of AIDS is Benjamin Freedman, in his "An Analysis of Some Social Issues Related to HIV Disease," below, pp. 93–104. Freedman's position is impaired, however, by his failure to distinguish between those who occasionally have homosexual sex and those who are "gay" as a regular way of life and who, from a halakhic point of view, are therefore "provocative sinners"; see below, p. xxvii, with n. 9.

11. In Conservative Judaism the question is under dispute. The chairman of the movement's Law Committee writes in a responsum: "I have issued an invitation or perhaps a demand to the halachically concerned homosexual to refrain entirely from homosexual practice by remaining celibate and by not engaging in the common homosexual lifestyle" (quoted by Schulweis, "Moral-

ity, Legality and Homosexuality," p. 8). As against this, Rabbi Harold M. Schul-weis of the Valley Beth Shalom Temple in Encino, California, follows a line of thought not unlike that of N. Lamm. In reaction to the just-quoted responsum he writes: "I confess that I cannot for the life of me look into their [homosexuals'] eyes and deny them intimacy, love, pleasure, and sensuality that is God's gift. . . . To bring misery, pain, torture, anguish to innocent people who are created the way they are violates my Jewish consciousness. . . . I do not regard these people as sinners or their love as abomination" (ibid., p. 9.).

12.   E.g., Rosner, "The Acquired Immunodeficiency Syndrome (AIDS)," pp. 178–179; idem, "AIDS: A Jewish View," below, p. 41; idem, "Rabbi Moshe Feinstein's Influence on Medical Halachah," p. 19; Novak, "The Problem of AIDS in Jewish Perspective," below, p. 77. Cf. also, more broadly: Brayer, "Drugs: A Jewish View."

13.   Freundel, "AIDS: A Traditional Response," below, pp. 24f.

14.   Ibid., p. 27. This point is emphasized by Rabbi Freundel in the "Postscript: Ten Years Later," added to the reprinting of his original 1986 article in this volume; below, p. 35.

15.   I am grateful to Rabbi Barry Freundel for having made his position clear to me in private correspondence.

16.   Indeed, until about 1986–87, the public religious discourse on AIDS in the United States was dominated by popular preachers who declared AIDS to be God's judgment on gays and other sinners; during that period the mainline Christian denominations did not officially take a position on AIDS, leaving the public space solely to demagogic preachers. See Shelp and Sunderland, *AIDS and the Church*, pp. 15–16. On fundamentalist positions on AIDS as an expression of divine wrath, see Kowalewski, "Religious Constructions of the AIDS Crisis," p. 93; idem, *All Things to All People*, p. 24; and for an overview, Altman, *AIDS in the Mind of America*, pp. 65–70, and Rushing, *The AIDS Epidemic*, pp. 171–173, 201–202. In 1987, a poll indicated that 43 percent of respondents agreed that AIDS represented a "divine punishment" (*New York Times* October 11, 1987, p. I-18; quoted in Rushing, *The AIDS Epidemic*, p. 173). The notion that AIDS was a divine retribution was expressed (in 1984) even by a faculty member of an American school of medicine and published as an editorial in the *Southern Medical Journal*; see Rushing, *The AIDS Epidemic*, pp. 185–186.

17.   "In reality, the question of God's role in the AIDS epidemics is an issue of practical concern only as a result of the fundamentalist Christian–gay community split. For the Jew, it is of no more than secondary or tertiary importance when compared to the practical issues raised by the spread of AIDS. In fact, the question of divine retribution, regardless of how it is resolved, affects no difference in the way the Jew is to respond to the present situation." Freundel, "AIDS: A Traditional Response," below, p. 27.

18.   Ibid., p. 25.

19.   Ibid., p. 26.

20.   Freundel to Freudenthal, January 11, 1996.

21.   Freundel, "AIDS: A Traditional Response," below, p. 26.

22. Ibid., p. 26.

23. Ibid., p. 26, with reference to TB *Ketubot* 30a and the Tosafot ad loc., s.v. *hakol bi-yedey*.

24. Ibid., p. 26.

25. Ibid., pp. 26f.

26. For a good brief overview, see the *Encyclopaedia Judaica* (Jerusalem, 1972), 13:1279–86, s.v., "Providence."

27. Indeed, as will be seen immediately below, David Novak qualifies this view as one that "most moderns" consider to be "an ancient superstition long behind us."

28. Freundel, "AIDS: A Traditional Response," below, p. 27.

29. Novak, "The Problem of AIDS," below, p. 75.

30. Ibid., p. 75.

31. Ibid., p. 76.

32. Ibid., below p. 76 and p. 88, n. 5, with reference to Exod. 20:5 and 34:7, Num. 14:18, Deut. 5:9.

33. Ibid., p. 78.

34. Ibid., p. 88, n. 4, with reference to TB *Berakhot* 33a and parallels re Deut. 10:12.

35. Jakobovits, "Halachic Perspectives on AIDS," below, p. 14. Rabbi Jakobovits had expressed this view very clearly already in 1986 in his celebrated article in *The Times*: "Both at the individual and the public level, we are certainly never entitled to declare a particular form of suffering as a punishment for a particular manifestation of wrongdoing. We can no more divine why some people endure terrible ills without any apparent cause than we can comprehend why others prosper though they clearly do not deserve their good fortune." Jakobovits, "Only a Moral Revolution," below, p. 2.

36. Jakobovits, "Only a Moral Revolution," below, p. 2.

37. Ibid., p. 3.

38. Jakobovits, "Halachic Perspectives," below, p. 15.

39. Ibid., p. 14.

40. Ibid., p. 15.

41. Jakobovits, "Only a Moral Revolution," below, p. 3.

42. Ibid., p. 3.

43. [Jessurun], "Le sida: réflexions juives," p. 10.

44. Steinberg, "*AIDS—Hebetim*," p. 86.

45. Bleich, "AIDS: A Jewish Perspective," p. 55. Similarly, Dr. Abraham Steinberg, who contrary to the authors discussed so far is a medical practitioner, writes unambiguously that viewing the AIDS victims as "having brought the disease upon themselves by immoral or illicit behavior" is "morally unacceptable, since a direct cause-and-effect relationship between sinful life and AIDS cannot and should not be ascribed by ordinary people"; see Steinberg, "AIDS: Jewish Perspectives," below, p. 62 ("*AIDS—Hebetim*," p. 84).

46. Bleich, "AIDS: A Jewish Perspective," pp. 52–53. An identical statement is made by Dr. Abraham Steinberg in his "AIDS: Jewish Perspectives," below, p. 166 ("*AIDS—Hebetim*," p. 84).

47. Bleich, "AIDS: A Jewish Perspective," p. 55.

48. Ibid., p. 56.

49. Ibid., pp. 55–56.

50. "Report of the Ad Hoc Committee on Homosexuality and the Rabbinate," adopted by the Central Conference of American Rabbis, June 25, 1990 (mimeographed).

51. Resolution adopted by the 97th Annual Convention of the Central Conference of American Rabbis, Snowmass, Colorado, June 26–30, 1986, § 4; below, p. 166.

52. The statement is taken from a synopsis of a presentation made by Rabbi Joel Roth, chairman of the Committee on Jewish Law and Standards, at a plenary session of the Biennial Convention of the United Synagogue of Conservative Judaism, November 15–19, 1987, Kiamesha Lake, New York, but does not represent the official position of the Committee on Jewish Law and Standards. It is quoted from *AIDS: A Jewish Response. For the Synagogues of the Conservative Movement. A Manual for Synagogue Leaders*, rev. ed. (New York: United Synagogue of Conservative Judaism, September 1994), p. 3. The official resolutions on AIDS of the Rabbinical Assembly (Conservative) that I have examined (5747–1987; May 1, 1991) and of the United Synagogue of Conservative Judaism (1987, 1991) do not explicitly refer (positively or negatively) to the doctrine of divine retribution. (These resolutions are reproduced below, pp. 159–163.)

53. See above, n. 16.

54. Viewing AIDS as a natural outcome of sinful conduct that perturbs the natural equilibrium of the cosmos is a position held also by some conservative Christian writers. Patrick Buchanan, notably, wrote in the *New York Post* of May 24, 1983, that the homosexual way of life is a declaration of war on nature and that through AIDS "Nature is fighting back" (quoted in Rushing, *The AIDS Epidemic*, p. 171). The underlying idea here too is that of a natural equilibrium that has been disturbed through homosexuality. To be sure, Buchanan's aggressive rhetoric is altogether absent from the writings of the Jewish thinkers we have studied. See also Kowalewski, "Religious Constructions," p. 93; idem, *All Things to All People*, p. 24.

55. Cf. Kowalewski, "Religious Constructions of the AIDS Crisis."

56. Kowalewski, *All Things to All People*, pp. 47–53.

57. "When the [Christian] denominations speak officially, the notion that HIV/AIDS is punishment for specific sins is rejected"; Shelp and Sunderland, *AIDS and the Church*, pp. 28f. For an overview of the attitudes adopted by the various Christian denominations, see ibid., pp. 20–30.

58. Zion, "AIDS and Homosexuality," p. 23.

59. Thus the Roman Catholic bishop William E. Swing, episcopal diocese of California, has written: "When I read about Jesus Christ in Scriptures and try to understand something of the mind of God, I cannot identify even one

occasion where he pictures his Father as occasionally becoming displeased and then hurling epidemics on nations. . . . Thus I do not believe in the God who becomes displeased and decides to show his anger by murdering large number of people, or in this case homosexual people" (William E. Swing, "Open Letter to the Reverend Charles Stanley," January 18, 1986, unpublished, quoted from Shelp and Sunderland, *AIDS and the Church*, p. 24). Similarly, Bishop John Roach of St. Paul and Minneapolis writes: "What a terrible question. Is AIDS the work of God? You know and I know that can't be true. That is not the way God's love and mercy shows itself among people" (Quoted from Melton, *The Churches Speak On: AIDS*, pp. xviii, 41; cf. pp. 4, 16). Again, a document of the Evangelical Lutheran Church in America, dated 1986, argues: "Gay and lesbian people with AIDS have been accused by some Christians of suffering the wrath of God for their sexual orientation. Such accusations are repulsive and contrary to the gospel of Christ. The presence or absence of disease can never be used as a theological benchmark for God's attitude toward any specific individual. One need only think of Job, whose suffering led his friends to question his righteousness, to recognize that this attitude was already challenged in the wisdom literature of the Hebrew Scriptures. . . . An observation about the state of health of an individual can no more be a measure of God's favor than an observation about one's bank account can be a measure of God's graciousness in business affairs. . . . Underlying the accusation that AIDS patients suffer God's specific wrath is a form of moralism about homosexuality which, in essence, supplants the gospel. Once a group is identified as more 'sinful' than others (implying, of course, that the accusing group is more righteous), sin becomes relativized and the radical character of God's grace is subverted" (quoted from Melton, *The Churches Speak On: AIDS*, p. 83). For various analogous statements, see Melton, ibid., pp. 127– 128, 131, 136, 143–144, 175, and Alizari, *Bioethics*, p. 295. An exceptionally sustained argumentation against the "wrath-of-God theory" is found in a study published by the Methodist Church of the United Kingdom (1987); cf. Melton, op. cit., pp. 101–104.

60. Cf. e.g. Jakobovits, *Jewish Medical Ethics*, pp. 131–134 (with extensive bibliography) and Rosner, "Visiting the Sick."

61. Jakobovits, *Jewish Medical Ethics*, pp. 69–74.

62. Rosner, "AIDS: A Jewish View," below, p. 43.

63. Numbers 17:6–15.

64. Freundel, "AIDS: A Traditional Response," below, p. 28. The same argument is adduced, independently it would seem, by B. Freedman ("An Analysis of Some Social Issues," below, p. 96). Freedman also adduces the following, only apparently analogous instance: "Moses's sister, Miriam, is struck with leprosy as punishment for having spoken ill of him; he prays for her recovery" (ibid., referring to Numbers 12:13). To adduce this instance as relevant to the issue under consideration is fallacious, however: Moses *prayed*, rather than *acted physically*, in order to avert the illness. Taking this instance seriously as relevant would imply that it is only through God's pardon that a sufferer (who contracted an illness as a punishment for a sin) can hope to be

healed; the physician's (or anyone's) role would be limited to praying for the sufferer. Adducing this text is thus strictly counterproductive!

65. Novak, "The Problem of AIDS," below, p. 78.

66. Ibid., p. 79, referring to TB *Mo'ed Qatan* 5a and Maimonides, *Hilkhot Tum'at Zara'at* 10:8.

67. Rosner, "AIDS: A Jewish View," below, p. 43, referring to BT *Sanhedrin* 73a.

68. Ibid., p. 43; Steinberg, "*Mahalot. AIDS,*" p. 600, n. 300.

69. As will be seen, however, Rav Deichowsky construes PWHIVs and PWAs as *rodefim*, or at least as potential *rodefim*. Obviously this view can be used to justify any restrictive measures against PWHIVs and PWAs; specifically, it would seem to entail that there is no obligation (or that it may even be prohibited) to extend medical help to them; see below, p. xxxix.

70. Rosner, "AIDS: A Jewish View," below, p. 43. See also Rosner's letters to the editor, *Journal of the American Medical Association (JAMA)*, Nov. 18, 1988 (vol. 260), pp. 2837–38 and April 21, 1989 (vol. 261), p. 2199.

71. Steinberg, "AIDS: Jewish Perspectives," below, p. 62 ("*AIDS— Hebetim,*" p. 84).

72. Bleich, "AIDS: A Jewish Perspective," 54. Similarly, the British Orthodox Rabbi Alan Unterman writes: "Whatever the attitude of traditional Judaism to the sexual activities of gay people, and however much some Jews may disapprove of Jewish gays, this does not affect their status as Jews, albeit Jewish sinners." Unterman, "Judaism and Homosexuality," 7.

73. For obvious reasons, this question is not at all an issue for Reform Judaism, which treats it as a social question on a par with any other. Cf. the Statement adopted by the Executive Board of the CCAR in June 1990 (this volume, 166f.). It includes e.g. the following: "Be is further resolved that we call upon our colleagues to take all necessary steps so that each community in which they serve has in place outreach to Jewish persons with AIDS and to their loved ones; i.e. pastoral care, funding for those in need, alternative medical care systems, etc." Conservative Judaism similarly urges that all help and assistance be extended to PWHIVs and PWAs. The resolution passed at the Convention of the Rabbinical Assembly, March 29–April 2, 1987, at Atlanta, Georgia, for instance, states (this volume, 162): "Be it resolved that we, the members of the Rabbinical Assembly, in convention assembled, demonstrate our compassion to all those affected: patients, parents, partners, families and friends; and declare that all *mitzvot* making manifest Judaism's love of all human beings and Judaism's compassion for the sick appertain hereto with full force, including such areas as *bikkur holim*; and decry all unjust discrimination in such areas as medical attention, housing, insurance and education."

74. Freedman, "An Analysis of Some Social Issues," below, pp. 96f., referring to Exodus 15:25 and TB *Nedarim* 41a. David Novak somewhat similarly argues that according to Judaism all humans are mortal because they are sinners; see "The Problem of AIDS," below, p. 78. Similarly, Dr. Abraham Steinberg writes that viewing AIDS as a divine retribution would lead to abstaining

from treating many patients "because there is no death without sin, and there is no righteous man on earth who does not sin." Steinberg, "*AIDS—Hebetim*," p. 84 (modified in "AIDS: Jewish Perspectives," below, p. 62).

75. See, e.g., the discussion in Deichowsky, "Compulsory Testing and Therapy," below, pp. 105–108 ("Kefiyat Bediqah we-Tippul," pp. 28–30). Cf. Steinberg, "*Arba'a Turim* of Jacob ben Asher"; Rosner, "AIDS: A Jewish View," below, pp. 42ff.

76. Novàk, "The Problem of AIDS," below, p. 80, referring to TB *Avodah Zarah* 26b.

77. Ibid.

78. The same consideration would seem to apply to the suggestion recently put forward by Rabbi Hillel Goldberg: "God measures each violation of the ritual, ethical, character and attitudinal norm not only, nor even primarily, against its objective magnitude, but against the magnitude of the subjective struggle necessary to prevent it. The stronger the inherent drive toward the violation, the greater the Divine mercy toward the violator. The weaker the inherent drive toward the violation, the more severe the Divine judgment of the violator." The upshot of this view is this: "the religious norm, however onerous, is retained without compromise; God's acknowledgement of the pain of those unable to keep the norm is also retained without compromise." (Cf. Hillel Goldberg, "Homosexuality: A Religious and Political Analysis," quotations from pp. 30-31.) It would seem that Goldberg's view, just as Lamm's, may be considered as risky in that it can be interpreted as offering a principled toleration ("mercy") of a constantly reiterated breach of a divine norm. Goldberg's position makes homosexuality into an entirely private affair, for, obviously, an individual's degree of struggle and pain cannot be known but by him/herself and by God. This implies that society must willy-nilly accept, or at least tolerate, homosexual conduct, except where it is openly claimed to be an alternative, permissible, life-style. Goldberg's position thus denies society any judgmental faculty in normative matters, because they involve unobservable facets of one's inner life (struggle, guilt feelings, etc.).

79. As noted earlier (p. xlviii, n. 10), B. Freedman ("An Analysis of Some Social Issues," below, p. 96) follows N. Lamm in arguing that homosexuals should be considered as falling under the category of *ones*. He fails, however, to distinguish between those who are regular homosexuals and those who have homosexual sex only occasionally. But *ones* can be claimed only for the former group, because those belonging to the latter obviously *are* able to abstain from homosexual sex. Freedman's argument therefore breaks down: those who are occasional homosexuals cannot claim *ones*; and those who are strictly gay are necessarily "provocative sinners," whom most thinkers, as just noted, refuse to consider as acting under *ones*, for fear that this may lead to accepting homosexuality as a legitimate way of life. Nor can Freedman's following suggestion be upheld: "[even] in the absence of excusable psychological compulsion [i.e., in the absence of the assumption of *ones*], reasoning from the status of the act [as sin] to that of the actor [as a sinner] is impossible

because of the possibility that the actor repented" (ibid., p. 96). In fact, most homosexuals, especially those whom Halakhah must regard as "provocative sinners," ostensibly do not repent. (The argument from repenting is adduced, as Freedman notes, in the case of suicide; the obvious difference is that in that instance, indeed, the actor's repentance can be assumed without the risk of contradiction.)

80. Novak, "The Problem of AIDS," below, pp. 82–83.

81. Rosner, "AIDS: A Jewish View," below, p. 44; emphasis added.

82. He writes: "Even when the illness is the result of homosexuality or drug addiction, and *particularly* when these transgressions are done out of desire and not provocatively (*le-hakh'is*), we are obligated to do our best also for AIDS patients"; Steinberg, "*AIDS—Hebetim*," p. 84 (emphasis added; somewhat abridged in "AIDS: Jewish Perspectives," below, p. 62). Note that the halakhic difficulty involved in justifying help for a provocative sinner is carefully avoided.

83. Cf. Kahn, "Le sida et ses incidences sur la Halakhah," p. 26. This report contains no detailed discussion: it merely states that the case of an occasional (homosexual) sinner (*le-te'avon*), who should not be judged and to whom help must be extended, is "totally different" from that of a provocative sinner (*le-hakh'is*) who acts by "ideological opposition to the Torah." The practical meaning of this phrase seems to be that in Israel Jews who die of AIDS and who are known (or presumed) to have been gays are at times denied a grave within the cemetery proper, and are buried beyond the cemetery's limits.

84. Thus Dr. Fred Rosner writes: "At the same time that we condemn homosexuality as an immoral act characterized by the Torah as an abomination, we are nevertheless duty bound to defend the basic rights to which homosexuals are entitled. The Torah teaches that even one who is tried, convicted and executed for a capital crime is still entitled to the respect due to any human being created in the image of God. Thus, his corpse may not go unburied overnight. The plight of Jewish AIDS victims doomed to almost certain death should arouse our compassion." Rosner, "AIDS: A Jewish View," below, p. 55.

85. Johnson, "Model of Factors."

86. Douglas, Kalman, and Kalman, "Homophobia Among Physicians and Nurses"; Kowalewski, *All Things to All People*, p. 23, referring to Altman, *AIDS in the Mind of America*; Orr, "Legal AIDS," p. 61; cf. the comprehensive account in Horsman and Sheeran, "Health Care Workers and HIV/AIDS."

87. "In New York, a minister said he was in a religious catch-22: He wanted to show concern and compassion for AIDS patients, but there are definite biblical injunctions against homosexuality. 'How,' he asked, 'can I support these people without supporting homosexuality?'" Quoted in Stine, *Acquired Immune Deficiency Syndrome*, p. 349.

88. Bayer, "AIDS and the Gay Community," p. 589. Popular preachers opposed the spending of tax-money on research on the "gay-disease" construed as a divine punishment; cf. Shelp and Sunderland, *AIDS and the Church*, pp. 19, 23.

89.   As indeed it was by the compilers of Melton, *The Churches Speak On: AIDS*, who saw fit to emphasize that while on the issue of homosexuality the three main branches of Judaism are divided, by contrast "on the issue of AIDS, the community seems to have developed a consensus view which calls for compassion towards people with AIDS and protection of their civil rights" (p. 165; cf. also pp. 166, 168, 169).

90.   The fact that an early survey, conducted in 1985, found that practicing Jewish health-workers experienced somewhat less homophobia with respect to their AIDS patients than practicing Catholics can perhaps be taken as an empirical confirmation of this thesis (Douglas, Kalman, and Kalman, "Homophobia Among Physicians and Nurses," p. 1310). The survey is admittedly of limited scope, but may well reflect global tendencies.

91.   Rosner, "AIDS: A Jewish View," below, pp. 45f.

92.   Ibid., p. 46.

93.   E.g., Freundel, "AIDS: A Traditional Response," below, p. 29ff.; Steinberg, "AIDS: Jewish Perspectives," below, pp. 67ff. ("*AIDS—Hebetim*," pp. 88–89); Bleich, "AIDS: A Jewish Perspective," pp. 69–74.

94.   Novak, "The Problem of AIDS," below, p. 87.

95.   This point was not yet quite clear in 1986, when Rabbi Freundel wrote his article, whence his ambivalent position on the issue. Cf. Freundel, "AIDS: A Traditional Response," and the "Postscript: Ten Years Later," below, pp. 29ff. and 35.

96.   Rosner, "AIDS: A Jewish View," below, p. 46ff.

97.   The United Synagogue of Conservative Judaism and the Central Conference of American Rabbis mention *biqqur holim* in practically all their resolutions and in their teaching material on AIDS.

98.   Cf. Washofsky, "AIDS and Ethical Responsibility," and the debate that this article has triggered. *Journal of Reform Judaism* 36, no. 3 (Summer 1989): 85–87; 36, no. 4 (Fall 1989): 80–81.

99.   See, e.g., *Nishmat Avraham*, vol. 4, *Even ha-'Ezer* § 2 (A.2), pp. 182f. (reprinted in Halperin, *An International Colloquium on Medicine, Ethics & Jewish Law*, pp. 184–185). In July 1993, Joshua Neuwirth, an ultra-Orthodox Jerusalem rabbi, opined that when husband or wife are seropositive, the use of a condom in order to safeguard the marriage may be permissible. This opinion was qualified as "a bomb" by Dr. M. Halperin, the director of the Falk Schlesinger Institute for Medical-Halakhic Research at the Shaare Zedek Medical Center in Jerusalem. See the account in *Ha'arez*, July 16, 1993, p. B-7. A similar view is expressed by Rabbi J. D. Bleich in his "AIDS: A Jewish Perspective," pp. 68–69.

100.   Jakobovits, "Memorandum on AIDS," below, pp. 8f. On the historical and political context of Rabbi Jakobovits's "Memorandum," see Berridge, *AIDS in the UK*, pp. 135–137. Berridge comments that Rabbi Jakobovits was the only religious leader to express opposition to the British government's AIDS campaign (although he at the same time commended the campaign for its urgency and for "striking the right balance between hysteria and complacency"); ibid., p. 137.

101. Jakobovits, "Only a Moral Revolution," below, p. 4.

102. Ibid., p. 4. Dr. Abraham Steinberg, in his comprehensive survey of Orthodox positions on problems related to AIDS, refers to this stance with approval. Cf. Steinberg, *"Mahalot. AIDS,"* p. 597.

103. Jakobovits, "Halachic Perspectives," below, p. 21 (cf. also p. 4).

104. Rabbi Sirat expressed his position in a statement to conference on "Religious Leadership in Secular Society," Jerusalem, February 1–4, 1994 (mimeo, p. 5). Reported in *Ha'arez*, Feb. 4, 1994, p. A-10. The same view was expressed by Rabbi Rivon Krygier (Conservative); cf. Rausky, "De la théologie du châtiment divin," p. 25.

105. Plaut, "'Saving Life as an Overriding Demand.'"

106. Jakobovits, "Only A Moral Revolution," below, p. 4. A similar position is expressed by Steinberg; cf. "AIDS: Jewish Perspectives," below, pp. 63f. (*"AIDS—Hebetim,"* p. 85).

107. Jakobovits, "Only a Moral Revolution," below, p. 3. In the article as printed in the *Times*, Isaac Arama is not named, but the reference is given in a privately distributed version (which is the one reprinted here); I am grateful to Lord Rabbi Jakobovits for having provided me with a copy of it.

108. Ibid., p. 3.

109. Steinberg, *"AIDS—Hebetim,"* pp. 87–88 (abridged in "AIDS: Jewish Perspectives," below, p. 66). The opposition within Jewish Orthodoxy between the more restrictive stance of Rabbi Jakobovits and Dr. Steinberg and the more liberal position of Rabbi Sirat is strictly paralleled in the Catholic Roman Church. The counterpart to the more liberal view is found in a document published in December 1987 by the administrative board of the U.S. Catholic Conference, entitled "The Many Faces of AIDS: A Gospel Response." The document, on the one hand, stressed that "the best source for prevention [of AIDS] for individuals and society can only come from an authentic and fully integrated understanding of human personhood and sexuality," with the consequence that "we oppose the approach often popularly called 'safe sex.' This avenue comprises human sexuality—making it 'safe' to be promiscuous." On the other hand, the bishops accept the idea that "educational efforts, if grounded in the broader moral vision outlined above, could include information about prophylactic devices or other practices proposed by some medical experts as potential means of preventing AIDS" (see Melton, *The Churches Speak On: AIDS*, pp. 25–27). Just as Rabbi Sirat was to do some years later, the bishops hastened to add that "abstinence outside the marriage and fidelity within the marriage . . . are the only morally correct and medically sure ways to prevent the spread of AIDS" (ibid., p. 27). In contrast, R. Jakobovits's position is identical with that of the conservative critics of the above-quoted document. Thus, Cardinal Joseph Ratzinger, prefect of the Congregation for the Doctrine of Faith in the Vatican, wrote (May 29, 1988), quoting and endorsing an article from *L'Osservatore Romano*: "'To seek a solution to the problem of infection by promoting the use of prophylactics would be . . . unacceptable from the moral aspect. Such a proposal for 'safe' or at least 'safer' sex—as they say—ignores

the real cause of the problem, namely, the permissiveness which, in the area of sex as in that related to other abuses, corrodes the moral fiber of the people'" (ibid., p. 34). In France, too, the Social Commission of the Episcopate has condoned the use of condoms, although it has underscored that their use cannot be the exclusive answer to AIDS; the response to AIDS should consist of a trilogy—the use of condoms, a limited number of sexual partners, and abstinence. See Commission sociale de l'épiscopat, *SIDA. La société en question*, pp. 156, 222, 231. Cf. Kowalewski, *All Things to All People*, pp. 29, 58, and Elizari, *Bioethics*, pp. 311–312.

110.   "Dans une situation de danger de mort, il faut préconiser l'utilisation de préservatifs. . . . Nous légiférons pour des situations illégales car bien évidemment les rapports sexuels hors marriage ne sont pas conformes à la morale du judaïsme." Reported in Rausky, "De la théologie du châtiment divin," p. 25.

111.   Rabbi Jakobovits's felicitous phrase "moral revolution" has caught on in Great Britain. Thus, only a few days after the appearance of Jakobovits's article in the *Times*, Cardinal Hume of the Roman Catholic Church published in the same newspaper (Jan. 7, 1987) an article entitled: "AIDS: Time For a Moral Renaissance" (Berridge, *AIDS in the UK*, p. 135). Similarly, early in 1987, Dr. Donald English, then Moderator of the Free Church Federal Council, said on a BBC broadcast: "I do not believe one minute that AIDS is God's direct punishment for sexual immorality, but I do believe that while sexual promiscuity didn't create AIDS there's now no doubt that it contributes enormously to its spread, with deadly consequences. Containing action won't remove AIDS: *a revolution in moral behaviour is needed* because we live in a moral universe." Melton, *The Churches Speak On: AIDS*, p. 104; emphasis added.

112.   Orr, "Legal AIDS," p. 63.

113.   "AIDS is the first worldwide epidemic to occur in the modern era of human rights. For the first time, public health practitioners are being held to a dual standard in the design and implementation of public health programs, in this case to prevent HIV transmission. Programs must be effective in public health terms, but in addition they must respect and respond to human rights norms." Mann, Tarantola, and Netter, *AIDS in the World*, p. 538. For a discussion of how the private and the public interests are reflected on the legal plane, see Orr, "Legal AIDS."

114.   See Bayer, "AIDS, Public Health, and Civil Liberties," for an insightful analysis of the way this balance has been struck in the United States.

115.   Mass screening for a large part of the population was initiated in Bulgaria, Cuba, and the former Soviet Union. At present (1996), Cuba is the only country pursuing this approach. However, many countries have abstained from screening not because of human rights considerations, but owing to the great cost and complex logistics of such a procedure. Cf. Mann, Tarantola, and Netter, *AIDS in the World*, p. 552. On the categories of persons subjected to selective screening in various countries, see ibid., pp. 553–558.

116.   Bleich, "AIDS: A Jewish Perspective," p. 59.

117. The most conspicuous case in point is the fetus that threatens its mother's life and whose life may, therefore, be taken; see Bleich, "AIDS: A Jewish Perspective," p. 60; also Jakobovits, "Halakhic Perspectives on AIDS," below, p. 17; Bleich, "Abortion in Halakhic Literature"; Sinclair, "The Legal Basis." It hardly needs mentioning that the notion of *rodef* became sadly famous following its abuse by the murderer of Israeli Prime Minister Yitzhaq Rabin in November 1995.

118. Bleich, "AIDS: A Jewish Perspective," p. 60.

119. Ibid. One may wonder why an analogous conclusion could not be reached apropos of the use of condoms by unmarrieds: why can it not be condoned by virtue of the general interest in saving lives? The reason is obviously that whereas individual rights are not anchored in Halakhah, so that following the "public good" does not collide with any halakhic imperative, the use of condoms, in contrast, is held to run counter to an explicit halakhic interdiction.

120. Ibid., p. 60.

121. Steinberg, "*AIDS—Hebetim,*" p. 87 (paraphrased in "AIDS: Jewish Perspectives," below, pp. 65f.).

122. "Sexual practices that offend morals and damage the health of the individual and the public are not beyond the scope of norms and laws. Consequently, homosexuality cannot be considered a private sexual conduct which is innocent, for it is strictly against the laws of the Torah." Steinberg, "*AIDS—Hebetim,*" p. 87 (abridged in "AIDS: Jewish Perspectives," below, p. 66).

123. Rabbi Bleich notes that Jewish Law incorporates a "hierarchical ranking of values" ("AIDS: A Jewish Perspective," p. 62).

124. Deichowsky, "Compulsory Testing," below, pp. 108–109 ("Kefiyat Bediqah we-Tippul," p. 31).

125. Deichowsky, "Compulsory Testing," below, p. 110 ("Kefiyat Bediqah we-Tippul," p. 32).

126. Cf. Jastrow, *Dictionary,* 1:215a; Elon, *Jewish Law,* 1:421–426, 436–439.

127. Deichowsky, "Compulsory Testing," below, p. 110 ("Kefiyat Bediqah we-Tippul," pp. 32–33).

128. This point is made (in another context) by David Novak: "AIDS is a disease, which at least for the time being, allows its sufferers only to be treated, not cured. No one's life, now anyway, can be 'saved.' We can only *care for* these lives in the little time they have left." "The Problem of AIDS in Jewish Perspective," below, pp. 86f..

129. Deichowsky, "Compulsory Testing," below, p. 109 ("Kefiyat bediqah be-Tippul" p. 32).

130. See, e.g., Horton, "Truth and Heresy About AIDS," p. 18: "The unfortunate truth is that clinical trials have often failed to support the biologically plausible assumption that it is never too early to treat people. . . . Several early studies were based on the notion that early treatment—when the patient was infected but free of symptoms—was the sensible and biologically plausible course. They seemed to indicate that intervention in symptom-free or early symptomatic stages of HIV infection might be beneficial. However, in 1992 J.

D. Hamilton and his colleagues showed that AZT produced no survival benefit in patients with early symptoms. This result was followed by the devastating findings of the Anglo-French Concorde study group. In this, the largest and longest trial of AZT in HIV-positive men and women, early use of the drug conferred no advantages. Worse still, further studies have shown significantly more deaths in the group treated early." In fairness it must be added that at the time Rabbi Deichowsky was writing (ca. 1989), it was thought that early thera-peutic treatment with AZT (which in the United States was approved for use in March 1987) could slow the course of the illness in asymptotic PHIV and in preventing the occurrence of *Pneumocystis carinii* pneumonia; see Mann, Taran-tola, and Netter, *AIDS in the World*, pp. 642–643 (Box 15.2).

131.   Rabbi Jakobovits too introduces the notion of *rodef* into the discussion of AIDS but on different presuppositions, so that his and Deichowsky's conclu-sions are not directly comparable. Jakobovits's discussion relates to a hypo-thetical situation—which in 1986 he had reason to consider as possible, but which we have since come to know to be counterfactual—in which AIDS could be transmitted under conditions of normal social contact, as it occurs, say, between children at school. Jakobovits holds that under such (menacing) con-ditions, all PWHIVs and PWAs would fall within the category of *rodef*. After emphasizing, just as Bleich does, that the *rodef* may be entirely faultless, Jakobovits says that "in respect of *innocent bystanders*, third parties, exposed to the risk of infection, then, those who deliberately or innocently pass on the infection would come within the category of '*Rodef*,' and society would be enti-tled to protect themselves against any such threats to their lives" (Jakobovits, "Halakhic Perspectives on AIDS," below, p. 17; emphasis added). Obviously, Rabbi Jakobovits's *rodefim* are not identical with those of Rav Deichowsky, who, writing in 1989, already knew perfectly well that HIV is *not* transmitted by casual social contact. Rabbi Jakobovits does not say whether, under the con-ditions that we now know to factually obtain, PWHIVs and PWAs should nonetheless be regarded as *rodefim* (AIDS is usually transmitted only in situa-tions which are symmetrical and consensual [sex, shared needles], so that there is not an active pursuer and a passive victim, and, moreover, which Jewish law views as illicit for both individuals involved [the purported pursuer and the potential victim]). It would seem, however, that Jakobovits's view presupposes that someone will be qualified as a *rodef* only if he or she threatens *innocent bystanders*. Since this is not the case with HIV transmission, it seems that Rabbi Jakobovits would not approve of Rav Deichowsky's undiscerning argumenta-tion.

132.   Jakobovits, "Halakhic Perspectives on AIDS," below, p. 18.

133.   Bleich, "AIDS: A Jewish Perspective," p. 62. Although the prohibition on *lashon ha-ra'* is Biblical, its significance has been underscored only relatively recently, through its codification by R. Israel Meir haCohen (1838–1933), who is generally referred to as the Hafetz Haim, after his book on talebearing by that name (for the source of the name, see Psalms 34:13–14). Sources on *lashon ha-ra'* are gathered in the English adaptation of *Sefer Hafetz Haim*, entitled

Guard Your Tongue, by R. Zelig Pliskin (New York, 1975). (I owe the above reference and information to a communication from Dr. Miriam Birnbaum of York University, Canada, on the Internet discussion group "H-Judaic Studies," dated April 29, 1996.)

134.   Responsum by Rav Yitzhaq Zilberstein (quoting Rav Elyashiv) dated Kislev 5752, privately circulated by Ha-Hug li-Refu'ah wa-Halakhah, Israel; I am grateful to Rav Henri Kahn of Jerusalem for having provided me with a copy of several of Rav Zilberstein's responsa related to AIDS. This responsum is summarized in Kahn, "Le sida et ses incidences sur la Halakhah," p. 26.

135.   In addition to the arguments mentioned above to sustain their ruling, Rav Zilberstein and Rav Elyashiv also rejected just the type of concern voiced by Rabbi Bleich, albeit only for the case that the PWA in question was a male prostitute. They argue that in this case, those who are at risk are in any event transgressors and it is not our business to save them from danger. The rabbinical authorities are obligated merely to issue a warning to the public stating in general terms that "God has prepared the Angel of Death for sinners who sin by prostitution" (Responsum, Kislev 5752).

136.   Bleich, "AIDS: A Jewish Perspective", p. 62.

137.   Ibid., p. 63.

138.   Ibid., p. 64.

139.   Ibid., pp. 78f., n. 14.

140.   Ibid., p. 64.

141.   Ibid., p. 65.

142.   Ibid., p. 66.

143.   See ibid., pp. 65–66: A physician who must choose between (a) attending to four patients whom he will *quite likely* save and (b) attending to a single patient who will certainly die if unattended, but who, with very intensive care, will *certainly* be saved, will unquestionably attend to the greater number, since the probability of saving four persons is weightier in the balance than the certitude of saving a single one (Bleich, "AIDS: A Jewish Perspective," p. 66; I have slightly modified the example given by Bleich so as to make it better highlight his point). During the Second World War, Winston Churchill was informed of an imminent Nazi air raid on Coventry, but decided not to take any defensive measures because this would have revealed to the enemy the fact that its military code had been deciphered. Churchill sacrificed a (great) number of lives *hic et nunc*, anticipating the saving of a (still) greater number of lives in yet unidentified future circumstances.

144.   Ibid., p. 66.

145.   Ibid., pp. 67–68.

146. In the early years of AIDS there were also the hemophiliacs. More recently, most PWHIVs and PWAs, mainly in Africa and Asia, contract the virus through heterosexual sex.

Bibliography

Altman, Dennis. *AIDS in the Mind of America.* Garden City, N.Y.: Anchor Books Doubleday, 1986.

Bayer, Ronald. "AIDS and the Gay Community: Between the Specter and the Promise of Medicine." *Social Research* 52, no. 3 (Autumn 1985): 581–606.

———. "AIDS, Public Health, and Civil Liberties: Consensus and Conflict in Policy." In *AIDS & Ethics,* ed. Frederic G. Reamer, pp. 26–9. New York: Columbia University Press, 1991.

Berridge, Virginia. *AIDS in the UK: The Making of Policy, 1981–1994.* Oxford: Oxford University Press, 1996.

Bleich, J. David. "Abortion in Halakhic Literature." In *Jewish Bioethics,* ed. Fred Rosner and J. David Bleich, pp. 134–177.

———. "AIDS: A Jewish Perspective." *Tradition* 26, no. 3 (1992): 49–80.

Brayer, Menachem M. "Drugs: A Jewish View." In *Modern Medicine and Jewish Ethics,* ed. Fred Rosner, pp. 242–251.

Commission sociale de l'épiscopat, Albert Rouet, président. *SIDA. La société en question* (Paris: Bayard Éditions/Centurion, 1996).

Deichowsky, Shlomo. "Kefiyat Bediqah we-Tippul—Hebetim Hilkhatiyim al Mahalat ha-AIDS" [Compulsory testing and treatment—halakhic perspectives on AIDS]. *Assia* 45–46 (vol. 12, nos. 1–2) (Tevet 5749): 28–33. Reprinted in *Sefer Assia,* ed. M. Haperin, vol. 7, pp. 73–78 (Jerusalem, 1993), and in *An International Colloquium on Medicine, Ethics & Jewish Law,* ed. M. Halperin. pp. 161–166.

Deichowsky, Shlomo. "Compulsory Testing and Therapy for AIDS." *Assia* 2, no. 2 (May 1995): 10–12. Abridged English translation of Deichowsky, "Kefiyat Bediqah we-Tippul [A revised version of this translation is reprinted in this volume, pp. 105–112.]"

Douglas, Carolyn J., Concetta M. Kalman, and Thomas P. Kalman. "Homophobia Among Physicians and Nurses: An Empirical Study." *Hospital and Community Psychiatry* 36, no. 12 (December 1985): 1309–11.

Elizari Basterra and Francisco Javier. *Bioethics*. Collegeville, Minn.: Liturgical Press, 1994. The Spanish original of this work was published in Madrid in 1991.

Elon, Menachem. *Jewish Law: History, Sources, Principles* (Hebrew). 3rd enlarged ed. Jerusalem: Magnes Press, 1988.

Freedman, Benjamin. "An Analysis of Some Social Issues Related to HIV Disease from the Perspective of Jewish Law and Values." *Journal of Clinical Ethics* 1, no. 1 (1990): 45–49. [Reprinted in this volume, pp. 93–104.]

Freundel, Barry. "AIDS: A Traditional Response." *Jewish Action*, Winter 5747 (1986–87): 48–57. [Reprinted in this volume, pp. 23–37.]

Goldberg, Hillel. "Homosexuality: A Religious and Political Analysis." *Tradition* 27, no. 3 (1993): 28–35.

Halperin, M., ed. *An International Colloquium on Medicine, Ethics & Jewish Law, Tamuz 5753–July 1993: A Collection of Essays*. Jerusalem, 1993.

Horsman, Janet M., and Paschal, Sheeran. "Health Care Workers and HIV/AIDS: A Critical Review of the Literature." *Social Sciences and Medicine* 41, no. 11 (1995): 1535–67.

Horton, Richard. "Truth and Heresy About AIDS." *New York Review of Books* 43, no. 9 (May 23, 1996): 14–20.

Huber, Joan, and Beth E. Schneider, eds. *The Social Context of AIDS*. Newbury Park and London: Sage, 1992.

Jakobovits, Immanuel. *Jewish Medical Ethics* (Hebrew). Translated from the English by G. Bat-Yehudah. Jerusalem: Mosad Harav Kook, 1966.

———. "Only a Moral Revolution Can Contain This Scourge." *The Times* (London), December 27, 1986, p. 20. [Reprinted in this volume, pp. 1–5].

———. "Memorandum on AIDS, Submitted by the Chief Rabbi to the Social Services Committee of the House of Commons [1987]." *Assia* 2, no. 1 (January 1991): 7–8. Reprinted in *An*

International Colloquium on Medicine, Ethics & Jewish Law, ed. M. Halperin, E43–E44. [Reprinted in this volume, pp. 7–10].

————. "Halachic Perspectives on AIDS." *Assia* 2, no. 1 (January 1991): 3–7. Reprinted in *An International Colloquium on Medicine, Ethics & Jewish Law*, ed. M. Halperin, E39–E43. [Reprinted in this volume, pp. 11–22].

Jastrow, Marcus. *A Dictionary of the Targum, the Talmud Babli and Yerushalmi, and the Midrashic Literature*. New York: Pardes Publishing House, 1950.

[Jessurun, Yizhaq]. "Le sida: réflexions juives sur une calamité universelle. Interview du rav Yits'haq Jessurun. - Marseille." *Kountrass* (Jerusalem): no. 52 (Iyar–Siwan 5755/May–June 1995): 9–13.

Johnson, Stephen D. "Model of Factors Related to Tendencies to Discriminate Against People With AIDS." *Psychological Reports* 76, no. 2 (April 1995): 563–572.

Kahn, Henri. "Le sida et ses incidences sur la Halakhah." *Kountrass* (Jerusalem): no. 52 (Iyar–Siwan 5755/May–June 1995): 25–27.

Kowalewski, Mark R. *All Things to All People: The Catholic Church Confronts the AIDS Crisis*. Albany: State University of New York Press, 1994.

————. "Religious Constructions of the AIDS Crisis." *Sociological Analysis* 51 (1990): 91–96.

Lamm, Norman. "Judaism and the Modern Attitude to Homosexuality." In *Jewish Bioethics*, ed. Fred Rosner and J. David Bleich, pp. 197–218. First published *Encyclopaedia Judaica Yearbook, 1974* (Jerusalem: Keter, 1974), pp. 194–205.

Mann, Jonathan, Daniel J. M. Tarantola, and Thomas W. Netter, eds. *AIDS in the World: The Global AIDS Policy Coalition*. Cambridge, Mass.: Harvard University Press, 1992.

Melton, J. Gordon, ed. *The Churches Speak On: AIDS. Official Documents from Religious Bodies and Ecumenical Organizations* Detroit: Gale Research, 1989.

Novak, David. "The Problem of AIDS in Jewish Perspective." In idem, *Jewish Social Ethics* (Oxford, 1992), pp. 104–117. First published in *Frontiers of Jewish Thought*, ed. Steven T. Katz, pp.

141–156. Washington, D.C.: B'nai B'rith Books, 1992. [Reprinted in this volume, pp. 73–91.]

Orr, Alistair. "Legal AIDS: Implications of AIDS and HIV for British and American Law." *Journal of Medical Ethics* 15 (1989): 61–67.

Plaut, W. Gunther. "'Saving Life as an Overriding Demand' (A Jewish Perspective)." In *Vth International Conference on AIDS*, p. 953 (abstract no. WFO 15). Ottawa, 1989.

Rausky, Franklin. "De la théologie du châtiment divin." *Tribune juive*, no. 1305 (December 1, 1994): 24–25.

Rosner, Fred. "The Acquired Immunodeficiency Syndrome (AIDS): Jewish Perspectives." In *Jewish Values in Health and Medicine*, ed. Levi Meier, pp. 171–184. Lanham, Md.: University Press of America, 1991. [Partly reprinted in this volume, pp. 135–138.]

———. "AIDS: A Jewish View." In idem., *Modern Medicine and Jewish Ethics*, pp. 49–63. Originally published in *Journal of Halacha and Contemporary Society* 12 (Spring 1987/Pesach 5747): 21–41. [Reprinted in this volume, pp. 39–58.]

———. *Modern Medicine and Jewish Ethics*. 2nd revised and augmented ed. Hoboken, N.J.: Ktav, 1991.

———. "Rabbi Moshe Feinstein's Influence on Medical Halachah." In *Medicine and Jewish Law*, ed. Fred Rosner, vol. 2, pp. 3–32. Northvale, N.J.: Jason Aronson, 1993.

———. "Visiting the Sick." In idem., *Modern Medicine and Jewish Ethics*, pp. 43–47.

———, ed. *Medicine and Jewish Law*, vol. 2. Northvale, N.J.: Jason Aronson, 1993.

——— and J. David Bleich, eds. *Jewish Bioethics* New York: Sanhedrin Press, 1979.

Rushing, William A. *The AIDS Epidemic: Social Dimensions of an Infectious Disease*. Boulder, Colo.: Westview Press, 1995.

Schulweis, Harold M. "Morality, Legality and Homosexuality." Privately circulated paper, written ca. 1993. Mimeo.

Shelp, Earl E., and Ronald H. Sunderland. *AIDS and the Church: The Second Decade*. Louisville: Westminster/John Knox Press, 1992.

Shilts, Randy. *And the Band Played On: Politics, People, and the AIDS Epidemic*. New York: St. Martin's Press, 1987.

Sinclair, Daniel B. "The Legal Basis for the Prohibition of Abortion in Jewish Law." *Israel Law Review* 15 (1980): 109–130.

Sirat, René Samuel. Statement to the conference "Religious Leadership in Secular Society." Jerusalem, February 1–4, 1994.

Steinberg, Avraham. "AIDS—Hebetim Refu'iyim, Musariyim, wa-Hilkhatiyim" [AIDS—medical, moral, and halakhic perspectives]. In *Sefer Assia*, ed. M. Halperin, vol. 7 (Jerusalem, 1993), pp. 79–91. Originally published in *Assia* 47–48 (vol. 12, nos. 3–4) (Kislev, 5790/1990): 18–30.

———. "AIDS: Jewish Perspectives." In *Medicine and Jewish Law*, ed. F. Rosner, vol. 2, pp. 89–102. English translation of a slightly modified text of Steinberg, "AIDS—Hebetim Refu'iyim, Musariyim, wa-Hilkhatiyim." [Reprinted in this volume, pp. 59–71.]

———. "*Arba'a Turim* of Jacob ben Asher on Medical Ethics." *Assia* 1, no. 1 (May 1988): 3–4.

———. "Mahalot. AIDS" [Diseases. AIDS]. In *Enciqlopediah Hilkhatit-Refu'it*, ed. A. Halperin, vol. 3 (Jerusalem, 5753/1992), pp. 581–614. Reprinted in *An International Colloquium on Medicine, Ethics & Jewish Law*, ed. M. Halperin, pp. 167–183.

Stine, Gerald J. *Acquired Immune Deficiency Syndrome: Biological, Medical, Social, and Legal Issues.* Englewood Cliffs, N.J.: Prentice-Hall, 1993.

Unterman, Alan. "Judaism and Homosexuality: Some Orthodox Perspectives." *Jewish Quarterly* 40, no. 3 (Autumn 1993): 5–9.

Washofsky, Mark. "AIDS and Ethical Responsibility: Some Halachic Considerations." *Journal of Reform Judaism* 36, no. 1 (Winter 1989): 53–65.

Zion, William P. "AIDS and Homosexuality: Some Jewish and Christian Responses." In *AIDS in Religious Perspective*, ed. William Closson James, pp. 19–42. Kingston, Ont.: Queen's Theological College, 1987.

Only a Moral Revolution Can Contain This Scourge (1986)

Lord Immanuel Jakobovits

I have delayed publicly expressing a view on the awesome menace of AIDS now hanging like a monstrous medieval plague over mankind, despite pressures from within my community and beyond to make some authentic Jewish pronouncement. This is due not merely to the fact that most authoritative Jewish statements on the moral issues were made thousands of years ago.

The earliest sources of Jewish law and morality are quite unambiguous. The Bible brands homosexual relationships as a capital offence (Lev. 20:13), and execrates any sexual licentiousness as an abomination, whether in the form of pre-marital "harlotry" (Deut. 23:18) or of extra-marital adultery (Lev. 20:10). Equally stern are the warnings of national doom consequent on any defiance of these principles: the land itself will "vomit out" peoples violating these injunctions (Lev. 18:28–29).

My hesitation in adding a Jewish voice to the many religious and moral statements already widely publicized, and worthy of endorsement, has been accentuated by the uncompromising nature of these biblical strictures. The difficulties go beyond the dilemma of choosing between soothing platitudes and unpalatable truths.

I am still racked by doubts on how to react to such a horrendous threat, how to address an age not exactly attuned to the puritan language of the Bible, how to transcend the perplexities which baffle medical and government experts, and how to present deeply held convictions without causing offence, panic, or disdain for the very teachings I espouse.

There are questions to which I simply know of no categorical answers. Some are practical: is it right to advocate "safe sex"? Or, should all citizens be subjected to screening tests to identify carriers, and if so, how is this information to be used? Some questions are theological: can a disease like this, patently discriminating against certain sections of society, be attributed to divine wrath, or altogether be adjudged in moral terms?

And some are purely human: how can one reassure without spreading complacency, warn without condescension or self-righteousness, and highlight the horrific without inducing immunity to shock by horror? Altogether, are habits and behavior susceptible to change by moral exhortation, by publicity campaigns, or even by medical information?

Inscrutable as the answers may as yet be, and rudimentary as may be our understanding of the long-term effects of AIDS and its spread, not to mention the prospects of halting its ravages, certain facts seem incontrovertible as a basis for some conclusions in the light of Jewish insights and moral principles.

Both at the individual and the public level, we are certainly never entitled to declare a particular form of suffering as a punishment for a particular manifestation of wrongdoing. We can no more divine why some people endure terrible ills without any apparent cause than we can comprehend why others prosper though they clearly do not deserve their good fortune.

Even less are we ever justified in being selective, subjecting some scourges to this moral analysis while exempting others (AIDS, yes; but earthquakes or floods or droughts, no). There is no such simplistic relationship between evil and misfortune, if only because there are too many exceptions. According to Jewish exegesis, the prophet Isaiah had his lips scorched because he sinned in saying "I dwell in the midst of a people of unclean lips" (Is. 6:5–6).

There is all the difference—even if the distinction is a fine one—between ascribing massive suffering to personal or social depravity as a divine visitation, and warning that such depravity may *lead* to terrible consequences. If I warn a child not to play with fire, and it ignores the warning and gets burned, the hurt is not a punishment but simply a consequence. If people recklessly indulge in infidelity and end up in the agony of a broken marriage, they suffer no vengeance; they simply pay the inevitable price for moral negligence or turpitude.

Public information campaigns should therefore be explicit and unequivocal: AIDS is the price we pay for the "benefits" of the permissive society which, helped by the pill, liberal legislation and more "enlightened" attitudes, has demolished the last defences of sexual restraint and self-discipline, leading to a collapse of nature's self-defence against degeneracy.

An even greater price in human misery than deaths from AIDS is being paid for violating the imperatives of sexual morality: the devastation of the family, with millions of casualties, especially among young people driven to vice and crime by the absence of a loving home.

The provision of condoms, condoning and facilitating sexual irresponsibility, is therefore hardly the answer, even if they temporarily reduce the transmission of AIDS. They would only increase the ravages of personal degradation and social disintegration. In any case, what has to be carefully weighed is individual safety against the erosion of public standards. The principle is illuminated in a striking precedent—Jewish law and thought must invariably search for guidance in earlier sources.

A leading 15th-century Spanish-Jewish scholar objected to the establishment of facilities for communally controlled prostitution to keep licentiousness from running wild—even if this objection meant failing to prevent married partners from committing the capital offence of adultery (as implied in the Ten Commandments, Judaism makes no difference between killing a person and killing a marriage). He argued that however culpable individual indiscipline is, its mitigation cannot be sanctioned at the expense of the slightest public compromise with the Divine Law.[1]

True, in Jewish law the saving of life overrides all religious precepts. But even this pro-life stance has three cardinal exceptions: forbidden liaisons, murder and idolatry are proscribed even at the cost of life. This, too, would seem to rule out recourse to any measures, such as condoms for unmarrieds, which would encourage indecent conduct, though the rule might be invoked to treat more leniently the distribution of clean needles for drug-abusers.

No less important than clean needles are clean speech, clean thoughts and clean conduct. What will be crucial is the cultivation of new attitudes calculated to restore reverence for the generation of life and the enjoyment of sexual pleasures exclusively within marriage. Nothing short of a moral revolution will in time contain the scourge.

The role of governments in achieving these objectives is admittedly limited. Morality cannot be legislated, nor can politicians and civil servants become preachers. But the administrators of our national affairs cannot remain morally neutral either, when the eventual cost may be counted in millions of lives.

Governments can help to refine human behavior—for instance by opposing any legislation liable to weaken the bonds between husband and wife or parents and children. Equally governments can, by the careful use of language in official speech and documents, eliminate from the common vocabulary the kind of euphemisms or misnomers that make perversions acceptable. I think of words like "gay" for homosexual, "heterosexual" for normal, "safe sex" for inadmissible indulgence, and "stable relationships" for unmarried couples.

The Jewish experience demonstrates that in the final analysis only spiritual power is invincible as a shield against lust. This is perhaps reflected in observant Jews, however addicted to smoking, finding the Sabbath prohibition against lighting a cigarette far more effective than the most alarming health warnings in securing complete abstention from smoking for one day in seven.

They have also discovered that a conscience so trained prevails even in the most intimate relations between husband and wife: the religious ban on any physical contract for some 12 days in every normal month, regularly rejuvenating the marriage through an iron self-discipline, achieves more than the most skilled marriage counsellor could in regulating the rhythm of love and longing, Natural urges can be bridled in submission to a higher law.

What is needed, then, is a massive campaign mobilizing government resources and citizens of all faiths and of none to strive for moral excellence, to avoid the arousal of passions in literature and entertainment, to extol the virtues of fidelity, and to promote the utmost compassion for those struck by a hideous killer as a result of failings which may not be theirs but the society's into which they were born, and which to ennoble is the charge of us all.

Every action to promote these ideals has now become a life-saving operation—including saving marriages as the sole legitimate origin of all human life.

Notes

1. R. Isaac Arama, *Akedat Yitzchak,* Gate 20.

Memorandum on AIDS* (1987)

Lord Immanuel Jakobovits

This memorandum deals specifically with the public response to the challenge of AIDS, with special reference to the Government campaign as projected through the media.

I realise of course that there will be many new complex moral problems to be faced beyond those to which I have addressed myself. They will concern, for instance, questions on compulsory testing, the identification of carriers, the right of insurance companies or employees to obtain medical data otherwise protected by confidentiality, the risks to life in experimenting on possible cures or vaccines, and numerous other such perplexities. I do not know how far the remit of the Committee includes considering such questions. Nor could I readily produce answers for which I could claim moral authenticity in the light of Jewish teachings. But I am prepared to probe into these issues if invited to give an opinion on them.

The Government is to be applauded on the urgency, boldness, and effectiveness manifest in its campaign. It appears to strike the right balance between hysteria and complacency, between alerting, even alarming, the population on the potentially awesome threat posed by the scourge, and reassuring citizens against undue panic which could lead to communal neurosis already widespread in the U.S.A.

It is also important to consider the possible effects of causing the "high-risk" groups to sense that they may be threatened by mounting discrimination in employment, education and social integration. Such a feeling, if allowed to become acute, could well encourage a sense of despair and resentment, breeding the desire to seek safety in numbers, even by deliberately spreading the contagion. The utmost care is therefore needed in dealing with the affected groups compassionately and with understanding, individually as well as collectively, so as to ward off the danger of major social tensions erupting into violence and other threats to the population at large.

On the other hand, I am disturbed by the general thrust of the publicity campaign, as epitomized by the slogan "Don't Die of Ignorance." Ignorance is not a fatal disease, and the real source of the danger through irresponsible behavior ought to be far more explicitly spelled out.

Of course, I appreciate that a Government cannot take a moral stance, particularly on an issue on which public opinion is widely divided, and which affects so delicately the most intimate human relations. I accept the need for moral neutrality. But I cannot accept anything which publicly condones or encourages immorality. The present campaign does.

By speaking of "safe sex" or "safer sex," and by advising on recourse on condoms "unless you are sure of your partner," the campaign officially accepts some form of extra-marital relations as the norm. This introduces into millions of perfectly moral homes, and especially of children and young people hitherto sheltered from exposure to indecency and marital faithlessness, notions that had been utterly alien and unknown to them. This itself is immoral, and may in time prove a source of major moral corruption for the very element of society most concerned to preserve its immunity to pernicious influences of this kind. The slant of the campaign also provides justification for deviations from moral norms for those who may have hitherto hooked on "casual sex" and promiscuous conduct with some degree of disquiet or even guilt. This, too, is immoral.

Altogether, in effect the campaign encourages promiscuity by advertising it. It tells people not what is right, but how to do wrong and get away with it—much like sending people into a contaminated atmosphere, but providing them with gas-masks and protective clothing. It quite wrongly assumes some inability to exercise self-control, which is clearly the ultimate answer to the spread of the affliction.

Equally worrying is the sense of false security promoted in the campaign. By creating the impression that condoms are an effective safeguard, one can ultimately only increase the danger. Neither are condoms absolutely reliable when used, nor are they always likely to be used in moments when passions are aroused. Condoms cannot replace self-discipline as a shield against infection, and any pretense to the contrary is dangerous in the extreme. By promising safety, the campaign would only increase the spread of AIDS in the long run.

Moral attitudes are clearly already undergoing some significant changes, as borne out in the latest Gallup Poll (commissioned by the Bradman Charitable Foundation and issued in February 1987). It shows that 74% of the sample (1,115 people aged 16 and over) agreed that the only way of avoiding AIDS was to stick to one faithful partner, whilst 96% wanted schools to warn children about the dangers of casual sex. The Government should not do anything to inhibit this trend or to impede its gaining momentum.

It should also be realised that far greater than the suffering and expenditure imposed by AIDS on society is the social damage and financial cost caused by marriage break-downs or "alternative lifestyle"—in particular the appalling predilection to crime, violence and drug-addiction among children raised in the absence of a loving home, as well as in terms of inefficiency, anxiety and sheer desperation while at work among people afflicted by marital failure or unhappiness. Apart from the astronomical economic cost of this drag on output and social services, the resultant depression in turn drives people to sexual adventures outside marriage which cannot but aggravate the incidence of AIDS. The public campaign should therefore be thoroughly revised and redirected towards emphasizing marital stability as the only "safe" norm. Encouragement should be given, if only by token contributions to marriage training and counselling agencies, to some intensive preparation for the responsibilities of marriage inside and outside schools, eventually as a prerequisite for marriage registrations, in much the same way as driving courses leading to successful tests are taken for granted as a condition for the issue of driving licences to prevent damage and injury through inadequate training or recklessness. Sex education at schools should be specifically geared to preparation for marriage, including the avoidance of pre-marital sex which cannot but undermine a subsequent marriage as an anti-climax.

At the same time, it is not enough for the positive aspects of the campaign to be more explicit to the point of encouraging fidelity in marriage (not "stable partners" which is a circumlocution for immoral non-marital relations). The negative aspects, too, need to be spelled out more directly. With all the publicity of statistics, the population does not know that 96% of AIDS victims are in the "high-risk" groups, and that these are made up overwhelmingly of homosexuals with the rest through promiscuity and drug abuse. These facts must not be concealed by suppression or be fudged by euphemisms. They are as essential in public enlightenment as the knowledge that the virus may be transmitted by unclean needles or infected blood.

In short, the campaign should say plainly: AIDS is the consequence of pre-marital sex, marital infidelity, sexual deviation and social irresponsibility—sacrificing enduring happiness for momentary pleasures, and putting selfish indulgence before duty and discipline. In today's climate of moral questioning and a greater readiness to revise personal "life-styles," the message will not go unheeded and the long-term effects in repairing the social fabric based on solid marriages may prove to be enormous in defending society against and far transcending the awesome ravages of AIDS.

*Submitted by the Chief Rabbi to the Social Services Committee of the House of Commons.

Halachic Perspectives on AIDS (1987)

‎כ״ב

Lord Immanuel Jakobovits

In trying to bring some Halachic perspectives to bear on AIDS and its ramifications, I see our role as Jews here at a three-fold level. First, we are Halachically under an obligation to promote all human beings to be subject to the *"Sheva Mitzvot B'nei Noach,"* to the seven Noachide commandments, the fundamental moral order which includes laws on sexual morality, on incest, on adultery, and on anything that constitutes a violation of those normal constraints within which we are perfectly entitled to exercise our sexual drive. There is, then, the obligation to do whatever we can to promote the understanding, the knowledge and the study of these laws, and the submission to them— this is part of a Halachic dictate laid down in the Rambam, in his Code of *Hilchot Melachim,* as a religious obligation: *"Lochuf et kol ha'olam"*—to compel, as far as we have it in our power to do so, the whole world to abide by these laws.

So to begin with, we are directly under a religious obligation to share our moral commitments with our fellow humans, beyond the confines of our own people.

Secondly, there is the element of *Kiddush Hashem* which is quite distinct and separate, that we ought to be seen as Jews to be in the forefront of the moral pioneering, ethical engineering, in fulfilling our national purpose, which is to blaze a trail of

11

moral advancement for the world. In the past, we have been conscious of this assignment and have contributed enormously to the enrichment of the human experience, in moral terms. Ideas which today are commonplace and taken for granted the world over, were initiated by our people. Concepts like brotherhood of man, social justice, human rights as we call them today—all of these are part of our Jewish heritage. After centuries and millennia of aloneness in the commitment to these values, they are only now beginning to be shared by the rest of the human family. We are charged to fulfill the promise as given towards the end of the blessings and curses in the Torah: "And all the nations of the world shall see that the name of the Lord is called upon you—*ki shem Hashem nikra alecha*," viz. that we live a Godly life, an exemplary life within our home life, our family life, with integrity, and moral values. This in itself is a second assignment given to our people, and therefore should give us a sense of urgency and importance in seeking to be heard and seen in any public argument that impinges on moral considerations. Whether on abortion, or on AIDS, or on anything that is of moral nature, we should be seen as Jews to play our due part to contributing to public enlightenment and to the elevation, the ennoblement, of public life and of the social atmosphere within which we live.

Thirdly, and above all, Jews owe it to themselves to know what their heritage has to say. We shouldn't have to learn from newspaper articles and from other faiths that have borrowed many of our moral concepts from us; we should not be dependent on absorbing and cultivating moral values from those who were themselves originally nourished, sustained and inspired by our Jewish education, that we turn out young people who have been to Hebrew classes, and sometimes to day schools, but who are utterly alien in terms of understanding Jewish teachings. And I think that this is one of the saddest comments on the failure and indeed bankruptcy of Jewish teaching on basic moral values relating to our present-day experience. This is catastrophic! We have failed! Yes, we do teach them about observances of different kinds relating to Sabbath and prayers and laws of kashrut—but to imprison Judaism in the kitchen, the

Synagogue, the cemetery, is doing violence to the very basis of Jewish teachings: and if you just leaf through the pages of the Tanach and the Prophets, you will see that very little space is given there to matters of ritual, and the bulk is given over to moral and social relations between man and man based on decency, honesty and moral values.

So, on all three scores, we are here under a direct challenge to participate, to enrich our own understanding and research into how we would respond to what is, after all, an unprecedented scourge that now menaces the entire human race. Perhaps not yet sufficiently appreciated is the scale of the calamity that threatens us. I am told that it is anticipated that, if the present trends are maintained for the rest of this century (which is another 14 years or so), it can be expected that the number of fatal casualties from AIDS will amount to more than the total number of dead in the two World Wars, in excess of 40 million— worldwide of course. So we are dealing here with a calamity of such enormity in terms of numbers, not to mention the suffering that goes with it prior to death, that it staggers the imagination. Moreover, it is, I suppose, the first time since the days of Noah's Flood that we have such a universal visitation of suffering. There were, in the Middle Ages, plagues in vast epidemics; but they were localised pockets of outbreaks that ravaged whole populations, and yet limited to different parts of Europe at one time, occasionally elsewhere, nothing like the universal plague that is now manifest in the depths of Africa, in the United States, in this country, in Europe and, alas, also in Israel. So the universality of the phenomenon in itself is something entirely unprecedented.

Now, I wish to make at least a passing reference to a sensitive aspect of AIDS, and its victims—and I think we ought to be clear about this. One of my criticisms of the Government campaign is precisely that it fudges the issue and tries to blur the facts that stare us in the face. 96%, I gather from medical literature to-date, of the fatalities so far from AIDS are to be found among the homosexual community, or among so-called "high-risk" groups. And it has spread beyond, and the dangers are great that the contagion will increase. But at the moment, it is clearly a highly selective form of visitation, and therefore obviously raises the most profound theological and moral problems of interpretation of cause and effect, of the role of the supernatural, of God, of Divine Justice and punishment.

I will merely say, as I put it in my article in *The Times*, that from my reading of Jewish sources, it would appear that under no circumstances would we be justified in branding the incidence of the disease, individually or collectively, as punishment that singles out individuals or groups for wrongdoing and lets them suffer as a consequence. We are not inspired enough, prophetic enough, we have not the vision, that would enable us to link, as an assertion of certainty, any form of human travail, grief, bereavement or suffering in general with shortcomings of a moral nature—especially our generation, living as we still do, in the immediate aftermath of the Holocaust, where millions of Jews were done to death with the most unspeakable brutality. We certainly should beware of ever identifying specific forms of grief, suffering, or anxiety with specific moral or any other shortcomings. It is not part of the Jewish doctrine of reward and punishment to so identify individual cases with individual experiences of great anguish. I therefore do not go along with, but on the contrary, strongly reject and oppose those preachers, or would-be preachers, who declare that it is Divine vengeance, that the wrath of God is being visited on those who deserve it because they live in the cesspools of evil. On the contrary, we should seek to stretch out whatever hand of help, of understanding, of solace, of compassion one can to sufferers, not to inflict, in addition to the agony through which they go, the additional humiliation and indignity and reproof of saying "you deserved it." This is utterly un-Jewish, and is utterly to be rejected. But having said that, we should at the same time add, that certainly we can see here that the particular visitation that now devastates people potentially by the million, is a consequence of a form of life that is morally unacceptable, and utterly repugnant to us.

It is one thing to speak of a consequence, and it is quite another thing to speak of a punishment. The illustration I used was if you warn a child not to play with fire, lest he gets burnt, and the child then gets burnt, then the burning may not be a punishment for not listening, but it certainly is a consequence. Likewise, I think until we make clear that AIDS is a consequence, we do not get to the root of it. I think we should declare in very plain and explicit terms indicating that our society violated some of the norms of the Divine Law, and of the natural law, and that as a consequence we pay a price, and an exceedingly heavy price. This certainly is Jewish doctrine. So there is a clear line of demarcation between punishment and consequence to be drawn. I need hardly spell out to an informed audience, certainly one that is likely to know the rudiments of Jewish teaching, that any form of sexual gratification outside marriage cannot be condoned by Jewish law. Whether this is pre-marital, or extra-marital, or whether this is altogether unnatural in the form of homosexuality—we utterly disapprove of this as an abomination. It is treated by Biblical law as a moral aberration that we cannot come to terms with.

Some argue that there are innate, instinctive, natural inclinations or aberrations which some of us are born with; they do not follow the norms of heterosexual love of most of the population. It is also claimed that a genetic condition can predispose towards an irregularity in the form of homosexuality. Therefore, it is argued that we have to accept this, it is a fact of life that this exists. We cannot accept this argument. One might as well say that it is only a natural drive, a natural urge, that accounts for any unusual or abnormal passion or instinct within us. So that, if a married man is suddenly attracted to someone other than his wife to gratify a sexual urge—can he then also claim that this is just a normal drive which should therefore be condoned or sanctioned? Yet we still will maintain the need for exercising self-control and discipline to prevent extra-marital relations. By succumbing to temptation because it is natural one could justify the breach of all the Ten Commandments. Killing a marriage, and killing a human being (murder and adultery) are placed side by side in the Torah because they are regarded as equally heinous. In other words, the fact that an act is natural does not make it any less abhorrent or criminal.

This is consistent with a very fundamental Jewish belief. We believe that we are created as human beings in order to master our lusts, our passions, our natural drives and urges. And that is precisely the uniqueness of man, that we are not to become the defenceless victims, slaves, to our instincts, surrendering to them. We have the ability within us to exercise the moral control that enables us to "discriminate between right and wrong," even if it is against our natural urges. And, just as we occasionally have to overcome the natural urge of hunger, by having to fast, which requires an act of self-discipline, or by abstaining from any number of normal pursuits that the constant exercise in self-discipline requires of us, so here also, the mere fact that some urge is natural is not an excuse for surrendering to it.

Now, let me turn to some more specific problems raised by AIDS in a Jewish context. The other day, I saw a disturbing article in an American orthodox publication dealing with some Halachic ramifications of AIDS.[1] Evidently reflecting rather more panicky public attitudes prevailing in certain parts of the United States than they do here, the author, a very respectable and erudite Rabbi, suggests that because of the danger that may be involved in passing on the contagion, those who are known to be carriers of the AIDS virus can be denied, and possible should be denied, the normal rites of *Taharah*, of purification on death by the Chevra Kadisha.

For the "*mis'askim*," the (usually volunteer) officiants of the Chevra Kadisha, cannot be expected to expose themselves to even the remote danger of catching it, therefore they can deny this precious and sacred entitlement to those who may be so affected. Similarly, the suggestion is made that if there are children who happen to be carriers (they can even be congenital carriers by birth as we now know), one would not only be entitled, but required to exclude them from Jewish schools, from Jewish instruction under public auspices for fear that they may transmit the virus to others.

From medical information as far as it is available to me, there is no justification whatsoever for either suggestion: therefore Halachically such a ban would not be warranted since AIDS cannot be passed on under the conditions mentioned here if normal precautions are taken such as by the members of the Chevra wearing gloves. Certainly, we would not want to contribute to creating a sense of public hysteria which may itself undermine the resilience of society to a situation as threatening as this. Of course, were it to be established by some future research that indeed such danger does exist, unless public measures are taken to exclude all forms of contact between those affected and others, then there would be no question that it would become a Halachic imperative to prevent this.

Such a situation would involve an important Halachic principle. If there were five people in a boat, remote from land, and one of them, it would be discovered, suffers from (let us say) the bubonic plague, which is highly contagious, threatening the lives of the other four, then he becomes in Halachah a "*Rodef*," a "pursuer." Now, a pursuer or an aggressor does not have to be guilty. He can be an innocent party; so long as he pursues someone else's life, he forfeits his life and may be killed to save his victim or victims. In other words, you may save an innocent life at the direct cost of the pursuer's, innocent or guilty, in the fulfilment of the normal Torah regulation on the law of "*Rodef*," of aggressor or pursuer. To prove that a party need not be guilty to be a pursuer, or to come within this category, I would refer to the ruling of the Rambam—who mentions it expressly as based on a passage in the Talmud which seems to imply this—whereby an unborn child threatening the life of the mother may be destroyed deliberately if necessary, because the child is a "pursuer." Although the child is certainly innocent—the child did not deliberately set out to threaten the mother's life—nevertheless, its claim to life is set aside because of its categorisation as a "*Rodef*," in order to save a life that is threatened, that is under attack. Accordingly, in respect of innocent bystanders, third parties, exposed to the risk of infection, then those who deliberately or innocently pass on that infection would come within the category of "*Rodef*," and society would be entitled to protect themselves against any such threat to their lives. So far the Halachah, at least in theory.

Whether this could ever be implemented in practice, merely from the point of view of social realities, I frankly cannot see.

There are, of course, also weighty counter-indications, such as the danger that AIDS sufferers may regard *themselves* as victims of "pursuit," and therefore intent on spreading the infection deliberately, thereby protecting their own lives by seeking safety in numbers. I do not think there are any ready-made answers on how to deal with unprecedented situations of these proportions. Other problems, too, are baffling and defy any definitive answers: for instance, whether, as widely advocated, we should increasingly think of compulsory testing of people to discover if they are carriers or not. Considering that the incubation period can extend up to eight years, and during that time the illness can be transmitted, when would one be subject to such test? And to whom would one communicate the result—the patient on whom one would thereby inflict a shattering trauma, or others who would then ostracize the patient or otherwise discriminate against him? All these are frightful questions for which no immediate and reliable answers can yet be found.

Other practical issues, too, cannot easily be resolved. Assuming we do have compulsory testing, what do we do with those identified as carriers? Make them wear labels? Or, as has already been suggested in some quarters, tattoo them in certain parts of their bodies to brand them with recognisable marks? This, again, staggers the human mind at the moment. Therefore I do not think that one should glibly and superficially reach out for answers that will require, first of all, the careful cultivation of a social conscience, of a moral conscience, in the world, before one can begin to find socially and morally acceptable answers to questions of this magnitude. But, Halachically, the law certainly would be that those whose lives are in any way threatened have the right to take every measure to protect themselves under the law of "*Rodef.*"

I now come to my final and main point. My major criticism of the current campaign, as I expressed it the other day to the Secretary of State for Health, Norman Fowler, is that we are too readily prepared to promote the second best, instead of in the first instance advocating the ultimate and ideal solution. I have read in *The Jewish Chronicle* what Jewish young people are supposed to think: the overwhelming majority of views, as recorded in the interviews held, seemed to be that one cannot expect young Jews and Jewesses today to live a truly clean life, to live an absolutely moral life according to Jewish doctrines of modesty and self-control; therefore one must come to terms with the fact that people will have pre-marital adventures and the like. I could not think of a greater slur on our young generation, a greater offense to the dignity and integrity of young people than to make such a genralised accusation, assuming the inability of young people to live up to what used to be the most treasured virtue of our Jewish heritage, and that is the sanctity and the stability of the Jewish home. I think we are underestimating the power of resistance and of resiliance or indeed even the capacity of society generally retracing its steps and going through some kind of a moral revolution. Nothing could be more defeatist than simply to surrender faith in the rising generation, believing that we can never restore the norms of decency by limiting any form of sexual intimacites within marriage exclusively.

    And as I reminded the Secretary of State, I have no doubt that at present, the damage done of to the fabric of society by the erosion of marriages—in terms of the number of misfits resulting from divorce, of young people being raised without a father and a mother, without the love and compassion with which they should be raised, plus the social irritations with their enormous cost to society, to the nation, incurred by broken homes and single parents—that damage is far greater, at the moment, than the damage done by AIDS. Marriage breakdowns cost the nation appreciably more than AIDS. Therefore the black cloud of this scourge may have its silver lining, as it were, challenging us to restore the respect for marriage—above all, by education, by properly training and preparing for marriage. The whole attitude requires a thorough revision. Currently, it is utterly irresponsible. We simply allow people to have a fling trying out one marriage, and if it does not work, tomorrow they will have another fling. The lightheartedness with which people enter into it, flows from not being prepared for the earnestness of it, and the responsibilities that are involved. If we could invest only a fraction of the resources that currently have to be spent on a colossal scale on looking after AIDS victims, if we could spend that on fortifying home life, we would probably contribute more to containing AIDS and help to overcome the tragedy that faces us.

Altogether, the campaign presently conducted over the media and by leaflets dropped into every home is in some respect misguided, and in others perhaps even counter-productive. The slogan "Don't die of ignorance" is completely misleading. Ignorance is not a fatal disease. People die of high-risk behaviour, not of ignorance. Moreover, the condom campaign in effect condones immorality.

Telling people "protect yourself against the consequences of doing the wrong thing" is just like saying to them "we will send you into a contaminated environment, but we will provide you with gas masks and with protective clothing so that nothing will happen to you." It is, I think, utterly irresponsible to say "go and do whatever you like, but we will give you advice on how to protect yourself against the consequences."

Worse still, the campaign may well give a false sense of security. Not only is the condom itself not always absolutely reliable, but in the end, when the moment of temptation comes, the lovers at the height of their passion will forget about the protection, and therefore relying on it will contribute to spreading this plague instead of containing it, as the campaign seeks to do. So the dangers are great, and the whole focus here may be wrong.

Let me conclude with a more general observation of some relevance to our situation. The Biblical record begins before and at the dawn of the Patriarchal period with a striking contrast. There was Noah, who lived at a time of universal corruption: "ki hishchit kol basar"—precisely the same kind of corruption that we encounter today—and he saw a whole world drowning and yet did not care. He built his own ark, safe for himself, but he did not pray for the world, did not work to prevent the spread of the contagion and looked on safely from the security of his shelter. That has to be contrasted, ten generations later, to Abraham, who also faced a city that was corrupt, Sodom. From this derives the word "sodomy" which is the very reference to what we are talking about. Abraham could not tolerate this. For him the city's doom was something that stirred his conscience. There was not a single Jew in Sodom: nevertheless, he pleaded against the destruction of Sodom. That is how Jewish history begins, because no Jewish heart can be indifferent to people suffering, deserved or undeserved, corrupt or not corrupt. When fellow human beings are in danger, we are to plead for them, to work for them, to have compassion, to extend our feelings of empathy to them.

Similarly, the very last message of the Biblical reading on Rosh Hashanah and Yom Kippur, the holiest days of the year, is the story of Yonah's mission to Nineveh. Here, a prophet of God is sent out from the land of God to a pagan city, Nineveh. Miles away from his own homeland, across the ocean he was told "go and warn the population" to ward off the doom that would be theirs. The erosion of moral values would eventually rob them of salvation. The prophet tried to deny his mission and escape from it. But he was eventually forced back to it because our responsibility extends to pagan cities just as much as to our own community. We cannot simply wash our hands and say "it is not our business and we are not concerned." That is the final and ultimate message of the whole of the High Holidays.

However, before that, the reading of the Law for Minchah on Yom Kippur before the Haftarah is read, is the passage from Leviticus dealing with sexual morality and immorality. How does that relate to Yom Kippur? What has this to do with Yom Kippur? Yom Kippur is the one day on which we must not have intimate relations even with our own wives, let alone with outsiders. The real Holy of Holies of life is how we conduct ourselves in the most intimate moments. We are to be aware that God watches us, not only how we deport ourselves outside, in public, but in the most intimate moments of our existence. Someone watches, and we are accountable. That is the final message of the Torah readings on Yom Kippur. It is of no value to go through the whole procedure of atonement on Yom Kippur, of reconciliation with God, spending a whole day in Sanctuary, if we are not first and foremost to have a "send-off message," as it were, of Yom Kippur, a message on inner cleanliness, on purity of thought and of mind, on the controls which sanctify us, and which make us different from the brutes. The very heart of the Jewish message is, as I have put it, that more important than clean needles are clean thoughts and clean conduct.

If we as Jews are not going to represent this message, if we are going to despair of rescuing a generation that is afflicted and faces a colossal calamity, if we are simply going to surrender faith that it can be done, then we are guilty of a betrayal of our own people, and by extension of our fellow men. I think an enormous opportunity, as well as challenge, faces us to vindicate our survival after 4000 years. For if we did not still have something unique to contribute to the betterment of the human condition, and to the elimination of vice and crime and immorality from the world, then we might as well bow out. We have not had such a bad run. 4000 years as a people, we have done pretty well. Other bigger peoples than ours have come and gone and joined the limbo of history. Unless we are still indispensable by making incomparable contributions to the advancement of the human order and the progress of the moral law, we have nothing further to do, and we should have no complaints if the world now would shed no tears over the disappearance of our people.

If, however, we do justify our continued existence, vindicating our claim to survival by still making ourselves indispensable, and creating something that used to be exemplary (even Goyim used to hold up the Jewish home and its stability as an example), if we do that, then maybe, we will merit once again the final conclusion of that verse: *"Vra'u kol amei ha'aretz ki shem Hashem nikra alecha u'yar'u mimekah"*—and all the peoples of the earth will see that the name of the Lord is called upon you, and they will have respect for you." We will regain that reverence, that awe, and that respect which will ultimately ensure our physical as well as spiritual safety. By virtue of our contribution to the moral integrity and physical safety of all human brothers, for whose well-being we care desperately, we will merit our own security and assure the fulfilment of our purpose.

Notes

The preceding is a revised transcript of an address to the Union of Jewish Students at Hillel House, London, 1987.

1.   Barry Freundel, "AIDS: A Traditional Response," *Jewish Action*, Winter 1986–87, pp. 49–57. (In this volume, below, p. 23–37.)

AIDS: A Traditional Response (1986)

𝒳𝒶

Barry Freundel

Not since the fear of contracting polio ended with the discovery of the Salk vaccine in the 1950s, and possibly not since the Black Plague in the Middle Ages, has society been gripped by the fear of a particular disease as it is today in its reaction to the AIDS epidemic. Horror stories (the disease is in fact called "The Horror" in Zaire),[1] the incurable nature of the condition (the criterion for declaring a cancer patient cancer-free is five years of negative pathology tests; no AIDS patient has ever survived that long),[2] the doubling of the reported cases every 9–12 months,[3] and the awful and slow deterioration of the health of the AIDS sufferer, have created a crisis atmosphere.

This has been accompanied by outbreaks of near-hysteria on the part of those who might, even potentially, have contact with AIDS victims. I, personally, know of one Orthodox man who was engaged in homosexual activity and wanted to begin psychotherapy with the goal of ultimately changing his orientation. Though he was willing to pay any reasonable price, a long list of mental health professionals refused to see him for fear of AIDS contagion. It actually took him more than six months to find a therapist willing to sit in the same room with him to discuss his problems. There was no indication that this individual had

AIDS, or that he had been exposed to it. His homosexual activity was enough to erect the barrier of fear.

Most prominent in the media have been stories of the strong negative reactions of parents concerned with their children's potential exposure to AIDS-infected students and teachers in public schools. Health professionals have also been caught up in this uncertainty and concern, with most insisting on the strictest anti-infection measures. Some have actually refused to treat AIDS patients out of fear of their own susceptibility to the disease.[4] Fueling the atmosphere of panic is the realization that cancer, previously the most feared of all illnesses, is, in some of its manifestations, merely a symptom of AIDS.[5]

Adding a further discordant note to the litany of fear, outrage and protest is the fundamentalist Christian claim that AIDS is God's wrath visited on homosexuals and drug users for their "sins."[6] The effect of this assertion, according to "gay" spokesmen, is that the disease is not treated as seriously by the health industry as it would be had it infected the general population. Therefore, say these spokesmen, research dollars are not adequately appropriated, and care is limited to preventing the spread of the disease to the straight (both sexually and morally) community.[7] This claim has been mitigated somewhat by the recent development of two or three drugs that seem to have a positive effect on the health of the AIDS sufferer.

To date, there have been no noteworthy published Jewish responses to the AIDS problem. Yet, this is an issue that begs for clarification and the application of the Torah principles to a very difficult and sensitive situation. What follows is an attempt to answer some questions raised by this crisis: Is AIDS an instrument of divine retribution? What are the implications if it is? Should youngsters and teachers with AIDS be excluded from classrooms? May health professionals who fear for their own safety refuse to treat AIDS patients? Finally, what are the responsibilities of public officials in a situation like this?

* * *

To the question of AIDS as a divine retribution, no final answer can be given. We lack a prophet, *Urim we-Tumim*, or *Ruah ha-Qodesh*, to ask the One who knows. But evidence can be brought, on both sides of the issue, from our tradition.

By far the greater evidence indicates that God's retribution plays a role in epidemics such as AIDS. It would far exceed the province of this paper to cite more than a few of the large number of sources that deal with the role played by divine retribution in this world. What follows, then, is only a small, but hopefully representative, sample of Biblical and Rabbinic comments relevant to the discussion.

Perhaps the most familiar of the Biblical sources on the subject are the verses in the second paragraph of *Qeri'at Shema'* (Deut. 11:16–17) that promise God's strong negative response as the wages of sin. Coupling these verses with the awesome retribution described in the Biblical section known as the *Tokhehah* (Levit. 22:14–46, especially v. 37, and Deut. 28:15–68, especially v. 61) and with the Biblical prediction of the land's physical rejection of those guilty of immorality in general, and homosexuality specifically (Levit. 18), it does not take a great leap of faith to see the hand of God in the AIDS epidemic. (Admittedly, "the land" in this last source refers to the Land of Israel. But in the light of other sources cited here, and the many prophetic pronouncements that speak of God's judgment against Gentiles and their homelands [e.g., Amos 1:1–2:3], this detail may be overlooked.) Adding credence to this view is the fact that AIDS, in keeping with the simplest interpretation of the verses cited here, seems to have come from nowhere to attack groups openly engaged in immoral activity.

Many Rabbinic statements also reflect the view that God's divine punishment does play a definitive role in the affairs of contemporary man. One particularly dramatic statement is the midrashic discussion of the reasons for the destruction of the generation of the flood. The section reads:

ר' הונא בשם רב יוסף אמר: דור המבול לא נימוחו מן העולם. עד שכתבו גמוסיות לזכר ולבהמה. וכו'

Rav Hunah said in the name of Rabbi Joseph: "The generation of the Flood was not eradicated from the world until they wrote *gamusioth*[8] for men [homosexual relationships] and beasts." R. Simlai said: "Wherever one finds immorality, there one finds *androlepsia*[9] entering the world [from Heaven] and it kills the good and the bad." R. Azariah and R. Jehudah b. R. Simon said in the name of R. Joshua b. Levi: "For all [sins] the Holy One, may He be blessed, extends His anger, except for immorality" . . . [10]

These comments seem to be a frightening foreshadowing of the AIDS phenomenon.

Only a bit less dramatic, but equally significant, are the sources that speak of God arranging events—the collapse of a building, for example, or a drowning—so that those guilty of capital crimes which merit stoning or strangulation in a religious court, will receive the appropriate punishment. According to the Rabbis, this occurs in cases where the court is unable to function for lack of evidence,[11] or because, historically, religious courts with the authority to try such cases no longer exist.[12]

These few sources are representative of the vast majority of traditional statements on the subject that speak with unequivocal belief in the power and contemporary reality of divine retribution. All of these sources tend to support the "AIDS as Divine Retribution" theory.

On the other hand, a small number of sources seem to suggest a different approach. One is a Talmudic statement that seems to posit a certain randomness and human control in the spread of disease: "All is in the hands of Heaven, except heat, cold," and, presumably, the illnesses they bring.[13] It may be a bit of a stretch to apply this to the current AIDS situation, but some may wish to make this stretch.

A second statement of this type is one authored by the Hazon Ish in which he states that divine providence, as far as reward for leading the good life and punishment for doing evil is concerned, is not publicly revealed in this era.[14] The context of this remark is important here. The Hazon Ish is arguing for lenient treatment of contemporary sinners, basing his appeal on this statement. Since divine reward and punishment are not as universally visible today as they once were, we cannot easily blame sinners for their sins. Therefore, we should be more understanding of them, and reach out to them with "ropes of love" (עבותות של אהבה) and without unpleasantness. Given the context, one can possibly apply this comment to the AIDS situation and suggest that God is not merely using AIDS to punish sinners.

Finally, we should make the point that God's understanding of things is not the same as ours, and, therefore, we can ascribe causality in the divine realm only with great temerity, if at all.

It is hard, in an emotionally charged atmosphere such as we presently face, to look at the evidence objectively. As a result, a final determination on the question cannot, and perhaps should not, be made. However, the singling out of the homosexual and drug-user populations as victims of the disease does seem to point to, at the very least, a divine "cease and desist" order. Whether or not direct divine retribution is involved, Jewish tradition would certainly ask the AIDS sufferer, those at risk, and all who are touched by the disease, to take the appearance of the illness to heart. All involved should examine their deeds and repent for their sins.

This approach is not unique to the AIDS crisis. According to our tradition, a similar response could be evoked in anyone suffering from or touched by *any* illness.[15] This type of soul-searching and redirection of lifestyle may actually be happening as a result of the AIDS epidemic, even if not *"lishma"*—for the sake of Heaven.[16]

* * *

In reality, the question of God's role in the AIDS epidemic is an issue of practical concern only as a result of the fundamentalist Christian–gay community split. For the Jew, it is of no more than secondary or tertiary importance when compared to the practical issues raised by the spread of AIDS. In fact, the question of divine retribution, regardless of how it is resolved, affects no difference in the way the Jew is to respond to the present situation.

This statement is made in light of the story of Moses' actions when confronted with an incontrovertibly divinely originated plague (Numbers 17:6–15). The incident begins with the Jewish people criticizing Moses and Aaron for their handling of the rebellion of Korah and his band (Numbers 16). In the aftermath of Korah and his band being swallowed up by the earth, the Jews accuse Moses and Aaron of having killed "the people of

God." God is so angered by this specious charge that He responds by sending a plague to destroy the Jewish people.

The Torah records Moses' response as: "And Moses said to Aaron, 'Take the fire-pan and put in it fire from the altar and incense, and carry it quickly to the congregation and atone for them, for the anger has gone out from God.' And Aaron took, as Moses commanded, and he ran into the midst of the assembly and behold, the plague had started among the people, and he put the incense and atoned for the people. And he stood between the dead and the living, and the plague ceased" (vv. 11–13).

Whether the incense and the atonement would work on AIDS patients is, unfortunately, a moot question. Clearly, however, this Biblical story of a divine plague brought as divine retribution parallels the most extreme view of the AIDS situation. The authentic Jewish response consisted of trying to save as many people as possible. The same response should apply in the AIDS crisis, regardless of its origin.

Most compelling in this regard is the scene of Aaron running to atone for the people. One does not expect an individual of Aaron's age and stature[17] to engage in such undignified activity. (This is the only time in Biblical literature that Aaron is described as running. The one comparable incident is Abraham's running to greet and then to serve the angels [Gen. 18:2 and 7]; *hakhnasat orhim*, like *piqquah nefesh*, is important enough that one's dignity is suspended in the face of one's duty.) Lives were at stake and Aaron did all he could, as quickly as he could, to save as many people as he could.

This source speaks in unequivocal terms to the AIDS situation. It makes no practical difference if AIDS is divine in origin or not. Divine retribution is God's business—healing is man's. If God wants to punish someone, He can arrange for the punishment. He needs no support from me. If I am confronted with dangerously ill AIDS patients, my only agenda, as was Aaron's, is to heal them as quickly as possible: לא תעמד על דם רעך—"Do not stand idly on the blood of your neighbor" (Levit. 19:16) applies even when God is the source of danger. The question of AIDS as God's retribution may be of some philosophical import, but it has no practical implications for the community. Our task is to heal and prevent death wherever possible.

Moving to more specific questions, we will deal first with the issue of casual contact with AIDS sufferers (not blood or body fluids) and the fear of contagion. One who has blood and body fluid contact with AIDS sufferers is clearly at risk.[18] This type of contact is unequivocally forbidden by Jewish law (see below for sources on the prohibition against putting oneself in a clearly dangerous situation).

* * *

Despite media reports to the contrary, there seems to be a question of danger in casual contact with AIDS victims. Doctors in the field to whom I have spoken are not completely sure how the disease is transmitted.[19] Local *hevrot qadisha* will not do *taharah* on an AIDS victim because the doctors with whom they have consulted will not give unequivocal assurance that contagion will not result. In addition, there does exist a small, but significant, percentage of AIDS sufferers who do not fit the high-risk categories and for whom the question of how they contracted the disease remains very much a mystery.[20] Furthermore, in early April 1986, reports appeared in the media confirming that the AIDS virus can survive outside the body. The *New York Times*[21] also reported on the case of a child who contracted the disease from a parent. It is assumed that this child was born with this disease, but this is not absolutely clear.

It is hard to say how significant the danger of contracting AIDS from casual contact actually is. It may be very near zero. It is certainly far less than 50%, but how much less is unclear. The difficulty in analyzing the risk factors is compounded by the five-year-long incubation period of the disease and the consequent difficulty in identifying its source in some patients.[22]

To analyze the situation in halakhic terms, we begin with our tradition's response to different degrees of danger. Where there exists a clearly significant danger, there would be no question that contact would be forbidden.[23] A significant danger, in cases like this, includes even one which is substantial, but less than 50%. Danger of this magnitude is a matter of halakhic concern sufficient to require avoidance.[24] Even performance of a mitzvah

does not mitigate against the danger if the danger is well established (דקביע היזקא).[25] On the other hand, were there virtually
no level of danger, fear of the disease would be irrational and
not acceptable as the determinant of our behavior.[26]

However, in the AIDS case, as the danger level is small, possibly real, and unclear, the subjective element plays the crucial
role for Halakhah. If people worry about the danger (certainly
the case with AIDS, where anxiety is only the smallest of the
reactions), then it enters the category of *safeq sakanah* and it is to
be treated with the greatest seriousness. In that case, the "civil
rights" of the sufferers, in terms of quarantines and similar measures, are simply not a consideration. Health and danger take
precedence. Obviously, the most humane possible situation
should be created for the victim. This is a natural derivation of
the commandment to love one's neighbor as oneself (Levit.
19:18). The Talmud specifically applies this verse to the situation
of a man convicted of a capital crime.[27] It should, therefore, certainly apply in this case as well, but people who shy away from
contact for fear of contracting AIDS are within their halakhic
rights.[28] Further, though an individual concern may not be valid
if the danger is extremely small, when an entire community
fears for an even vanishingly small danger, such as putting a
coin in one's mouth, it is to be avoided.[29] In our case, the
community is obviously concerned, and one may argue for personal avoidance on this basis alone.

On the other hand, particularly given the status of the AIDS
victim as the contemporary leper, any real human contact probably constitutes a mitzvah under the rubric of *biqqur holim*.[30] As
indicated below, performance of a mitzvah may be enough to
mitigate against minor concerns. However, the mitzvah of *biqqur
holim* is not specific enough to the particular patient to mandate
contact as it does in the health professional's case discussed
below.[31] After all, one can visit any sick person and fulfill the
biqqur holim requirement. By the same token, those who are not
afraid of contagion may, halakhically, have reasonable (not sexual or body-fluid exchange) contact with AIDS sufferers.[32]

One source that effectively illustrates these parameters is an
incident recorded in *Pe'er ha-Dor*, the biography of the Hazon

Ish. This work contains not only the story of the Hazon Ish's life, but it is also an important record of his halakhic decisions. One of the anecdotes in the book details the Hazon Ish's response to the question of violating the Sabbath in getting to a bomb shelter when the air-raid sirens sound during wartime.[33]

This is parallel to the AIDS case in that there is some danger to life and limb, but it is unclear how much danger. (The sounding of sirens may only be a test or a false alarm; the bombs may not fall here; and even if they do, the likelihood is that they will miss me.) Yet people are afraid. The Hazon Ish publicly permitted the violation of even Biblical laws in this situation. However, he himself did not take advantage of the *heter*. He was not afraid, so he chose to rely on God to protect him as he refrained from violating the Sabbath. If the danger had been clear and obvious, the Hazon Ish would have been in violation of a Biblical imperative: ונשמרתם מאד לנפשותיכם (Deut. 4:15). But as the danger was small and unclear, the subjective element of the individual's personal level of concern was determinant.

* * *

When one carries the question of contact with AIDS sufferers to the case of school children, one enters an additional area of halakhic concern. Our tradition insists that children not be placed in any danger, even a remote danger, while pursuing an education. The Talmud states that children may be taken from one school to another for the purpose of study.[34] However, they may not be made to pass over a river for this purpose, unless there is a completely sturdy bridge to cross. If the crossing is made over a plank, the child may not be taken, even if the education is better on the other side.

This last case speaks of a plank which presents only minimal danger for those who walk it. If it did present a real danger, the local authorities would be required to remove it,[35] and no one, not just school children, would be permitted to use it. Presumably, this is a plank that people use regularly. They are, obviously, not concerned with the danger. Despite this, children, the darlings of the law, cannot be put in such a situation.

This halakhic point is actually applicable to the AIDS crisis in two ways. Healthy children may face some risk from AIDS sufferers. This is especially true for young children, who tend to have a great deal of contact with one another. They also tend to cut themselves frequently, and blood has been definitely implicated in the transmission of AIDS (see above).

In addition, one must also be concerned about the child with AIDS. Close contact with other children invites infection. For a person with an impaired immune system, such as the system of an AIDS victim, this may be suicidal. In fact, the danger may be so great that the child and his parents would violate the standards of *piqqu'ah nefesh*, without even getting into the special case of school children.

Certainly, our hearts go out to children suffering from AIDS, and we should provide the best educational opportunities we can for such students—but not in the regular classroom. Education and even remote danger do not mesh halakhically, and should not be present in our education system.

* * *

One further point on educational settings that also has larger ramifications should be made. Halakhah demands a higher standard of safety in the public domain than in the private domain. At least two sources indicate this. The Talmud states that a hot coal in a public area may be extinguished on the Sabbath because of the potential danger.[36] On the other hand, a Rabbinic prohibition forbids doing this in a private area.[37] Similarly, a parapet around the roof of a private house may be built on *hol ha-mo'ed*, but only using *ma'aseh hedyot* (the work of an unskilled laborer), while a dangerous ruin may be removed from a public domain on *hol ha-mo'ed* even using *ma'aseh uman* (skilled labor).[38]

The reason for the distinction between public and private domains in the two sources is statistically obvious. A risk which is small enough to be acceptable on an individual basis becomes a dangerous certainty in a macrosystem. Put another way, a 100 to 1 chance may be a risk that I can halakhically accept upon myself because I can be reasonably confident that I will be spared. But in a city of a million people, 10,000 deaths will result from this activity if the statistics hold true. The civil authorities, who bear the responsibility for society as a whole, therefore, cannot take the same risk as the individual.[39] Consequently, the authorities cannot let AIDS students into classes even if adult individuals may choose to have contact with these unfortunates. By the same token, bath-houses and other similar locations— which probably should have been closed for other reasons— must now, certainly, be shut down. The concern for the public safety simply overrides any individual rights which may be involved.

* * *

Finally we come to the case of health professionals refusing to treat, or allowing their fears to adversely affect their treatment of, AIDS victims. We have already discussed the subjective element in responding to cases of possible danger for the general public. In contrast, as in the case of school children, the subjective element all but disappears for the health professional. This time, however, the removal of the subjective element leads to the opposite conclusion. Where neither the school child nor his parents acting on his behalf can subjectively accept the risk of contact with the AIDS patient, the health practitioner cannot refuse such contact. Such refusal would constitute a lack of faith in God's providence and in His justice. The health practitioner involved is performing a mitzvah when he treats a sick patient.[40] In the AIDS case, given the health practitioner's standard training in avoiding contagion, there is, at worst, only a vanishingly small chance of infection. It would, therefore, be inappropriate to doubt that God would offer protection from this remote danger in return for the meritorious act of tending to the sick.[41] A similar rationale is apparently the basis for the halakhic principle שלוחי מצוה אינן ניזוקין—"messengers travelling for the purpose of a mitzvah are protected from danger."[42] Another point that may be applicable here holds that restrictions on facing minor danger are suspended if it is necessary to face such danger to make a living. This is based on Deut. 24:15 and is fully articulated in the Talmud.[43] Particularly if the strict isolation protective measures that include capping, gowning, shoe-covering, and gloving are taken, as they are in many hospitals, the halakhic view would seem to be that health practitioners who refuse to help AIDS victims, or who give inadequate care, violate the biblical prohibition of לא תעמד על דם רעך—"Thou shalt not stand inactive by the blood of your neighbor" (Levit. 19:16).

* * *

Before concluding with a summary of specific halakhic points covered in this article, a general statement on the issue needs to be made. Gay rights groups have attempted to make the AIDS issue a civil rights issue, and a kind of acid test of one's "liberal" credentials. In Judaism's view, this is patently absurd. AIDS is a health issue, no more and no less. The halakhic questions are those that relate to all health issues. In the same way that the issue of AIDS as divine retribution has no bearing on the way that we deal with the questions discussed here, the issue of rights of a person involved in homosexual activity also has no place here. Both questions are extraneous to the core problem, and invoking these issues simply makes a dangerous medical situation that much more complex and harder to solve.

* * *

In summation, then, Halakhah treats AIDS as it would any other health issue. The crucial concern is the severity and degree of danger. As contact with an AIDS patient seems to present some medically undefined level of danger, individuals have the right to be concerned for their own health, and therefore may insist on quarantine. Because of the lack of clarity, and the lack of obvious danger, other individuals may choose to ignore the risks and trust that God will protect them. School children, the darlings of Halakhah, may not have AIDS sufferers included in their midst out of concern for both the infected and non-infected students. Furthermore, health professionals are duty-bound to have a modicum of faith in God, and they must competently and professionally minister to AIDS patients. Finally, whatever can be done to find a cure for the disease should be done as quickly as possible, keeping in mind that resources are limited and other life-threatening diseases require research as well.

The halakhic position in the AIDS crisis, as it exists today, once we cut through the extraneous rhetoric, is clear and eminently reasonable. Our task now is to encourage medical research that seeks a cure. At the same time, a prayer that God grant us wisdom to find a cure and end the fear and suffering would also be appropriate.

Postscript: Ten Years Later (July 1996)

My article "AIDS: A Traditional Response" appeared in 1986 and was one of the first, if not the very first, published Orthodox reactions to the pandemic.

It appeared at a time when even the mechanism of contagion was not entirely known. Obviously, any reference to a possibility of casual contagion is, by present scientific understanding, out of place, and the discussion of that issue in the article is inoperative, as is the concern for contagion in the classroom that was based on that issue. AIDS is transmitted by blood and body fluid contact, scientists tell us, and it is in circumstances where such exposure is a possibility that care must be taken. The risk-benefit discussion in the article applies only in those areas as well.

Second, though I meant to be agnostic on the question whether AIDS is G-d's punishment for homosexual behavior and/or drug abuse, and thought I succeeded, some readers see me as favoring the view that it is G-d's retribution. My position on this subject remains clear to me even if I have not communicated it well to others. I do not sit at G-d's right hand, and He does not communicate with me about His reasons for doing things. In the absence of such communication, one can only search the sources. What one finds are citations that point in either direction. I do not believe that G-d never brings illness as punishment. I similarly do not believe that G-d always brings illness as punishment. Frankly, the victim is the one required *lemashmesh be-ma'asaw* (to examine his deeds) and to decide whether his present circumstances are commensurate with his past actions, and to repent if he finds a connection. My central point was and remains that the question of whether AIDS is Divine retribution or not is G-d's business. Mankind has one obligation: to heal. If healing is impossible, then alleviating suffering, both physical and psychological, becomes the requirement.

I would add only one more comment. When historians will look back on our own society's treatment of AIDS, they will come to two conclusions. First, that we were very foolish and, second, that we were very lucky. AIDS is the only illness ever treated with civil rights, and many have died because we did not follow the usual patterns of response to sexually transmitted diseases (STDs). Mandatory testing and informing sexual partners had helped stem the tide of other STDs and would have helped here. Sadly, the incidence of other STDs also increased as these policies lapsed under the assault of AIDS civil-rights advocates. Our hierarchy of values simply went awry as the right to privacy overtook the preciousness of human life. Luck entered the picture precisely because AIDS is not a very communicable disease. If it were more aggressive, our refusal to follow what had previously been standard procedure would have been far more deadly. Perhaps the hand of G-d can be found here, as well.

Notes

1. A. G. Fettner and W. A. Check, *The Truth About AIDS: Evolution of an Epidemic*, 2nd ed. (New York: Holt, Rinehart & Winston, 1985).

2. Ibid., p. 229; *Newsweek* 106, no. 7 (Aug. 12, 1985), cover and p. 20.

3. Fettner and Check, *The Truth About AIDS*, p. 212; *Newsweek*, Aug. 12, 1985, p. 20.

4. Fettner and Check, *The Truth About AIDS*, p. xi, 229–233.

5. Ibid., p. 40.

6. Ibid., p. 247; *Newsweek*, Aug. 12, 1985, p. 20.

7. Fettner and Check, *The Truth About AIDS*, pp. 209–210, 252; *Newsweek*, Aug. 12, 1985, p. 21.

8. The Greek *ketubah* according to *Arukh*; coupling songs according to Jastrow.

9. A dangerous plague, according to *Arukh*; the right of reprisals, according to Jastrow.

10. *Genesis Rabba* 26:5; see also *Levit. Rabba* 23:9.

11. TB *Makkot* 10b; see also *Avot* 2:6.

12. TB *Ketubbot* 30a, *Sotah* 8b, *Sanhedrin* 37b. See *Sanhedrin* 58a that homosexuality is a capital crime for Gentiles, and Levit. 20:13 that homosexuality is a capital crime for Jews.

13. TB *Ketubbot* 30a; See also Tosafot ad loc., s.v. *hakol bi-yedey*.

14. *Yoreh De'ah* 2:16.

15. See Aaron Berakhia b. Moses of Modena, *Ma'avar Yaboq* 1:3.

16. See Fettner and Check, *The Truth About AIDS*, pp. 248–249; *Newsweek*, Aug. 12, 1985, pp. 21, 28–29.

17. Aaron was 85 years at this time—see Ex. 7:7 and *Seder Olam Rabba*, vol. 1 (Jerusalem, 1922), pp. 9, 125.

18. Fettner and Check, *The Truth About AIDS*, p. 179; *Newsweek*, Aug. 12, 1985, p. 24.

19. See also Fettner and Check, *The Truth About AIDS*, pp. 156–158, 166, 179, 197, 200–201, 204–208.

20. Ibid., p. 4; *Newsweek*, Aug. 12, 1985, p. 22, reports 6.5% of adult AIDS cases and 11% of children's cases as not being from the high-risk groups.

21. Feb. 6, 1986, p. B7.

22. Fettner and Check, *The Truth About AIDS*, p. 5.

23. Deut. 4:15; TB *Berakhot* 3a, *Shabbat* 32a, *Pesahim* 112a, *Avodah Zarah* 12b, and other Talmudic sources. Also Maimonides, *Yad, Hilkhot De'ot* 4:1, *Hilkhot Roze'ah u-Shemirat ha-Nefesh* 2, esp. 4–6; *Shulhan 'Arukh, Yoreh De'ah* 116.

24. See TB *Yoma* 84b, also *Hullin* 10a: "Danger is treated more stringently than that which is ritually forbidden," and Tosafot, *Niddah* 44a, s.v. *Ihu*.

25. TB *Yoma* 11a, *Kiddushin* 39b, *Hullin* 142a.

26. See *Responsa Hatam Sofer, Yoreh De'ah*, no. 338; and *Responsa Ahi Ezer* 1:23; but see Maharam Schick, *Responsa, Yoreh De'ah*, no. 244, that even a one-in-a-million chance is significant enough for concern.

27. TB *Pesahim* 75a, *Ketubot* 37a, *Bava Qamma* 51a, *Sanhedrin* 45a and 52b, *Sotah* 8b.

28. *Responsa Ahi Ezer*, loc. cit., and the source in *Pe'er ha-Dor*, below, n. 33.

29. TJ *Terumot* 8:3; *Hagahot Maimoniot, Hilkhot Roze'ah u-Shemirat ha-Nefesh* 12, no. 2.

30. This is based on *Perishah* on *Tur, Yoreh De'ah* 335, no. 3; the story of Rabbi Akiba, *Nedarim* 40a, and Rashi ad loc., s.v. *ke'ilu shofekh damin.*

31. See TB *Yoma* 39b–40a.

32. *Responsa Avnei Nezer, Even ha-Ezer* 81:3.

33. S. Cohen, ed., *Pe'er ha-Dor* (Bnei Braq, 1970), 3:183–184.

34. TB *Bava Batra* 21a.

35. Maimonides, *Sefer ha-Mitzvot*, negative commandment 298.

36. TB *Shabbat* 42a.

37. Maimonides, *Yad, Hilkhot Shabbat* 1:7 and 12:2.

38. Ibid., *Hilkhot Yom Tov* 8:6.

39. Cf. S. Boylan, "Hashash Sakanah le-Or ha-Halakhah," *Or ha-Mizrah* 32(1) (no. 112) (Tishrei 5744): 48–59.

40. Cf. J. David Bleich, *Judaism and Healing* (New York: Ktav, 1981), chap. 1, "The Obligation to Heal" (pp. 1–10), for different opinions on the source for this mitzvah.

41. Cf. *Turey Zahav* to *Orah Hayyim* 455, no. 3, based on Ecc. 3:5.

42. TB *Pesahim* 8a–b, *Yoma* 11a, *Qiddushin* 39b, *Hullin* 142a.

43. TB *Bava Mezi'ah* 111b–112a.

AIDS: A Jewish View (1987)

א״ה

Fred Rosner

Introduction

The acquired immunodeficiency syndrome (AIDS) has been described as this century's greatest health peril. Thousands have already died from the disease and there is no cure in sight. The emotional toll on patients with AIDS, their families, and their caregivers needs to be actively and aggressively addressed. The public hysteria should be alleviated by a well planned, coordinated, and implemented educational program involving not only health professionals but the mass media and press, which have in part fueled the public fear about AIDS. Prudent practices in health care and private industry workplaces have been suggested and should be followed. Governmental involvement in terms of increased AIDS treatment and research funding is sorely needed. Finally, public policy decisions need to be made with compassion and understanding and the conviction that this disease can be tamed and eventually overcome by a concerted effort of all parties concerned.

Homosexuality and Drug Abuse in Judaism

Ninety percent of all patients with AIDS are homosexuals or intravenous drug abusers. The Torah labels homosexual intercourse as an abomination[1] and ordains capital punishment for both transgressors,[2] though minors under thirteen years of age are exempt from this as from any other penalty.[3] This biblical directive is codified by Rambam:

> In the case of a man who lies with a male, or causes a male to have connection with him, once sexual contact has been initiated, the rule is as follows: If both are adults, they are punishable by stoning, as it is said, *Thou shalt not lie with a male*, i.e., whether he is the active or the passive participant in the act.[4]

The prohibition of homosexuality proper is omitted from the *Shulchan Aruch*, which omission reflects the virtual absence of homosexuality among Jews rather than any difference of views on the criminality of these acts.[5] The Torah only refers to incidents involving homosexuality in regard to the sinful city of Sodom[6] and in regard to the conduct of a group of Benjaminites in Gibeah, leading to a disastrous civil war.[7] Isolated cases are also described in the Talmud.[8]

Rabbi Jakobovits cites rabbinic sources for the strict ban on homosexuality that is included among the seven commandments of the sons of Noah: it is an unnatural perversion debasing the dignity of man, it frustrates the procreative purpose of sex, and it damages family life.[9] He concludes that Jewish law rejects the view that homosexuality is merely a disease or morally neutral.

Rabbi Barry Freundel has posited that Jewish law views the homosexual or drug addict as no different than a Sabbath desecrator or an adulterer.[10] He has no greater or lesser rights or obligations and deserves no special treatment or concessions. The term "homosexual," says Freundel, is inappropriate. We should refer to this individual as a person engaged in homosexual activity. The term is not a noun but an adjective. The Jewish community should, therefore, deal with the practitioner of homosexuality as a full-fledged Jew, albeit a sinner; he should be counseled and treated and be the concern of outreach and proper education.

The use of consciousness-expanding drugs such as LSD or other addictive substances is generally considered to be proscribed by the halachah. According to Rabbi Moshe Feinstein, the harmful effects of marijuana are among the reasons for prohibiting its use.[11] The same can be said about smoking in Judaism.[12] Certainly the abuse of narcotics and other substances by the intravenous and other routes is detrimental to one's health and, therefore, prohibited in Judaism, for the Torah instructs us not to intentionally place ourselves in danger: *Take heed to thyself and take care of thy life*[13] and *take good care of your lives.*[14] The avoidance of danger is exemplified in the biblical commandment to make a parapet for one's roof so that no one fall therefrom.[15] Hence, the smoking of marijuana and the abuse of intravenous narcotics, which constitute a danger and hazard to life, are considered pernicious habits and should be prohibited. The subterfuge of "it is no concern of others if I endanger myself" is specifically disallowed by Rambam[16] and the *Shulchan Aruch.*[17]

Jewish Legal Questions Relating to AIDS

Not only is the intentional endangerment of one's health or life by the use of intravenous drugs prohibited in Jewish law, but wounding oneself without fatal intent is also disallowed in the Talmud[18] and the codes of Maimonides[19] and Rav Joseph Karo.[20] Since most patients with AIDS are homosexuals and/or drug addicts, they are considered sinners, thereby raising a variety of Jewish legal questions. Should a Jewish drug addict who develops AIDS as a result of sinful activity be treated any differently than any other patient? Should the Jewish homosexual who develops AIDS as a result of "abominable" behavior be treated? Does Judaism teach compassion for all who suffer illness irrespective of whether or not the illness is the result of practices which Judaism abhors and prohibits? Should every effort be made to heal these patients or at least alleviate their pain and suffering? Is a physician or nurse or other health worker obligated to treat a patient with AIDS or other contagious disease if there is a risk that he may contract the illness from the patient? Should the Jewish community expend resources for AIDS research and treatment, since most such patients are sinners? Would not the resources be better allocated if spent for the health of law-abiding citizens? Can patients with AIDS be counted in a quorum of ten men (*minyan*)? Can they serve as cantors or Torah readers? Should they be given honors in the synagogue? Can a *kohen* with AIDS go up to the *duchan* and offer the priestly blessing? Can a patient with AIDS serve as a witness in a Jewish legal proceeding? Is a patient with AIDS to be given all the usual burial rites? Is mourning to be observed for such a patient? These and other halachic questions pertaining not only to AIDS patients but to sinners in general were addressed in two separate discourses delivered by Rabbi Hershel Schachter and Rabbi Moshe Tendler, both senior faculty members at Yeshiva University. The following discussion is based in part on those discourses.

Obligation of the Physician to Heal a Sinner

The physician's license to heal is based on the biblical phrase *and heal he shall heal*,[21] from which the talmudic Sages deduce that divine authorization is given to the human physician to heal.[22] In his biblical commentary, Rabbi Moses Nachmanides, known as Ramban, states that since the physician may inadvertently harm his patient, divine permissibility to heal was necessary to absolve the physician of responsibility for any poor medical outcome, provided he was not negligent. Other commentaries assert that since sickness is divinely inflicted as punishment for sin, divine permission to heal is required to allow a human physician to intervene and provide healing.

Maimonides expands the permissibility for the human physician to heal into an obligation or mandate based on the biblical commandment for restoring a lost object to its rightful owner[23]—if a physician is able to restore a patient's lost health, he is obligated to do so. If a patient dies as a result of a physician's refusal to heal him, the physician is guilty of shedding blood for having stood idly by.[24] A detailed discussion of the physician's obligation to heal in Judaism can be found elsewhere.[25]

G-d cherishes the life of every human being and therefore requires all biblical and rabbinic commandments except idolatry, incest, and murder to be waived in order to save the life of a person in danger (*piku'ach nefesh*). The Sabbath must be desecrated to save a human life.[26] But is the desecration of the Sabbath allowed and/or mandated to save the life of a sinner who is guilty of a crime such as homosexuality for which the death penalty might be imposed?

The Talmud[27] permits the killing of a pursuer (*rodef*) to prevent him from killing the person he is pursuing; the one who kills him has no sin because the pursuer is considered to be legally (halachically) like a dead man (*gavra ketila*). For the same reason, one may *not* desecrate the Sabbath to save the life of the pursuer if a building collapses on him and his life is in danger. The same is true of a person sentenced to death by the court (Bet Din) in that one may not desecrate the Sabbath on his behalf if his life is in danger because he, too, is halachically considered like a dead man. However, a sinner who has not been sentenced by the Bet Din is considered as a live human being. As a result, although he is a transgressor, all biblical and rabbinic commandments must be suspended to save his life. Therefore, it seems clear that patients with AIDS should be treated medically and psychosocially no differently than other patients, and physicians and other medical personnel are obligated to heal patients with AIDS. The Talmud clearly states that every life is worth saving without distinction as to whether the person whose life is in danger is a criminal or a transgressor or a law-abiding citizen.[28] In fact, the Talmud requires that one expend money from one's own pocket to provide whatever is necessary to save another's life.

Some contemporary writers raise the issue of the difference between a provocative sinner (*mumar lehachis*) and a lustful sinner (*mumar lete'avon*).[29] The Talmud rules that a provocative sinner is not to be helped but actually hindered (*moridin velo ma'alin*).[30] The commentary of Rashi there and the code of Maimonides interpret a provocative sinner to refer to one who habitually and willfully sins.[31] On the other hand, one who only occasionally sins out of lust or appetite is considered like one whose life and property are to be protected and carefully treated.[32] It would seem therefore that physicians and other health personnel have an obligation to care for patients with AIDS no differently than for other patients.

Danger to Medical Personnel Treating Patients with AIDS

Jewish law requires that if one sees his neighbor drowning or mauled by beasts or attacked by robbers, he is bound to save him.[33] Elsewhere the *Shulchan Aruch* rules that if one observes a ship sinking with Jews on board, or a river flooding over its banks thereby endangering lives, or a pursued person whose life is in danger, one is obligated to desecrate the Sabbath to save them.[34] The commentaries of *Mishnah Berurah* and *Pitchei Teshuvah* add that if doing so involves danger for the rescuer, he is not obligated to endanger his life because his life takes precedence over that of his fellow man.[35] If there is only a doubtful risk (*sofek sakanah*) for the rescuer, he should carefully evaluate the small risk or the potential danger to himself and act accordingly.

What should a physician do if his patient is suffering from a contagious disease which the physician might contract? Is the physician allowed to refuse to treat the patient because of the risk or the fear by the physician of contracting the disease? What if the risk is very small? What is the definition of *sofek sakanah*? If there is a 50 percent chance of the physician contracting the disease from his patient, halachah would certainly agree that such odds are more than doubtful and the physician would not be obligated to care for that patient without taking precautionary measures to protect himself. If he wishes to do so in spite of the risk, his act is considered to be a pious act (*midat chasidut*) by some writers, and folly (*chasid shoteh*) by others.[36] But if the risk is very remote, the physician must care for that patient because *the Lord preserveth the simpletons*.[37] This phrase is invoked in the Talmud in relation to the remote danger of conception in a minor child[38] and is discussed in great detail by Rabbi Moshe Feinstein in a lengthy responsum concerning the use of a contraceptive device by a woman in whom pregnancy would constitute a danger to her life.[39] Contraception, states Rabbi Feinstein, is permissible for *sofek sakanah* but not where the risk is extremely small. Rabbi Shneur Zalman of Lublin and Rabbi Chayim Ozer Grodzensky respectively discuss whether the above biblical phrase is invoked for a minor risk (less than 50 percent) or only for a very remote and rare risk.[40]

Rabbi Yitzchok Zilberstein discusses the case of a female physician in her first trimester of pregnancy who is called to see a seriously ill patient with rubella (German measles).[41] The physician is at 50 percent risk of acquiring rubella and possibly giving birth to a seriously defective baby (blind, deaf, or mentally retarded) or she may abort or have a stillbirth. Although there are no fetal indications in halachah which would allow abortion, Rabbi Zilberstein posits that halachah considers miscarriage to be a situation of *pikuach nefesh* and rules therefore that the female physician is not obligated to care for a patient with rubella.

The question as to whether or not a person is obligated to subject himself to a risk in order to save another person's life is discussed in great detail in several recent articles[42] and briefly summarized by Professor A. S. Abraham in an article on human experimentation.[43] The matter is related to the well-known difference of opinion recorded in the two Talmuds. The Jerusalem Talmud posits that a person is obligated to potentially endanger his life (*sofek sakanah*) to save the life of his fellow man from certain danger (*vadai sakanah*).[44] This position is supported by Rabbi Meir Hacohen[45] as cited by Rav Yosef[46] and by Rav Karo himself.[47] On the other hand, the Babylonian Talmud voices the opinion that a person is not obligated to endanger his life to save that of another even if the risk is small (*sofek sakanah*).[48] The ruling from the Jerusalem Talmud is omitted from the Codes of Rif, Rambam, Rosh, Tur, and Ramo.

The prevailing opinion among the various rabbinic sources seems to be the one cited by the Radvaz:[49] If there is great danger to the rescuer, he is not allowed to attempt to save his fellow man; if he nevertheless does so, he is called a pious fool; if the danger to the rescuer is small and the danger to his fellow man very great, the rescuer is allowed but not obligated to attempt the rescue, and if he does so his act is called an act of loving-kindness (*midat chasidut*). If there is no risk at all to the rescuer or if the risk is very small or remote, he is obligated to try to save his fellow man. If he refuses to do so, he is guilty of transgressing the commandment *thou shalt not stand idly by the blood of thy fellow man*.[50] This approach is also adopted by recent rabbinic decisors including Rabbi Moshe Feinstein and Rabbi Eliezer Yehudah Waldenberg.[51] Since the risk to physicians and other health personnel in caring for AIDS patients is infinitesimally small (less than a fraction of 1 percent), it follows that a physician is obligated under Jewish law to care for such patients.

The same logic is used to allow but not require healthy people to donate a kidney to save the life of a close relative dying of kidney failure. Most rabbis, including Rabbi Ovadiah Yosef, Rabbi Jacob Joseph Weiss, and Rabbi Eliezer Waldenberg, and others support this halachic position.[52]

Visiting Patients with Infectious Diseases Such as AIDS

It is a duty incumbent upon everyone to visit the sick, for G-d visits the sick[53] and we must emulate Him.[54] Rabbi Jakobovits points out that the question whether the duty to visit the sick extends to visiting patients suffering from an infectious or contagious disease was already answered with a qualified affirmative by the Ramo against the view of some later authorities who questioned the need to expose oneself to the hazard of contagion in the fulfillment of this precept.[55] Ramo holds that there is no distinction in respect of visiting the sick between ordinary and infectious diseases, with the sole exception of leprosy.[56] A recent reexamination of this question, continues Rabbi Jakobovits, leads one to the conclusion, based on several talmudic narratives,[57] that the ruling of Ramo applies only to an infection which would not endanger the life of the visitor even if he caught it, but that one is not required to risk one's life merely for the sake of fulfilling the rabbinic precept of visiting the sick, nor can anyone be compelled to serve such patients. Elsewhere Rabbi Jakobovits asserts that in practice, the view of Ramo did not prevail, and approval was expressed for the custom not to assign visitations of plague-stricken patients to anyone except specially appointed persons who were highly paid for their perilous work.[58] Rabbi Jakobovits also cites the seventeenth-century records of the Portuguese Congregation in Hamburg, which indicate that even the communal doctors and nurses were exempt from the obligation to attend to infectious cases and that the required services were rendered by volunteers entitled to special remuneration.[59]

Rabbi Jekuthiel Jehudah Greenwald states that if there is hope of healing the patient from his illness, one is obligated to visit and serve him even if there is a risk of contracting the disease, because, according to the Jerusalem Talmud, one is obligated to accept a small risk in order to save one's fellow man from a definite danger.[60] However, if there is no chance of saving the patient, one should not endanger one's own life by visiting the patient.[61]

The Talmud states that those sent to perform a religious duty do not suffer harm (*shiluchei mitzvah aynon nizakin*).[62] This rule is also codified in Jewish law but only where there is no danger involved for the person performing the precept.[63] Where there is prevalent danger (*hezekey matzui*), the rule may not apply and the person may be foolhardy to risk his life to perform the precept (*chasid shoteh*). However, if the risk is infinitesimally small, such as one in a thousand or less, the person should fulfill the precept.

The risk of contracting AIDS by visiting or touching the patient seems to be nil. No case of AIDS has yet been contracted by casual contact with an AIDS patient. The virus is only transmitted through the blood and by sexual contact. Hence, physicians are obligated to care for patients with AIDS and everyone is obligated to visit patients sick with AIDS. The only precaution one need take is to avoid sticking oneself with a needle used to draw blood from or give an injection to an AIDS patient.

Allocation of Resources for AIDS Research and Treatment

Some people claim that governmental and societal resources should not be devoted to AIDS research because the disease is self-inflicted. This approach is obviously invalid, because some patients acquire AIDS through no fault of their own, i.e., through blood transfusions as in hemophiliacs, or transplacentally as in infants born of AIDS mothers. Even if a disease occurs only in sinners, society is still obligated to expend resources to try and conquer the disease, and physicians are obligated to heal patients suffering from that disease. The Talmud clearly states that every life is worth saving without distinction as to whether the person whose life is in danger is a criminal or a law-abiding citizen.[64]

The problem of the allocation of the resources of society when money for health care and medical research is limited is discussed in greater detail elsewhere.[65] Similarly, physicians have to allocate their time and energy among their various patients, raising halachic questions such as the permissibility (or prohibition) for a physician to leave one patient to care for another, much sicker patient. This topic, however, is beyond the scope of this essay.

Can Patients with AIDS Be Counted as Part of a Minyan?

May patients with AIDS who are homosexuals and/or drug addicts be counted as part of a quorum of ten men (*minyan*)? The *Shulchan Aruch* states that a sinner who transgresses the decrees of the Jewish community or who commits a biblical or rabbinic transgression can be counted as part of a *minyan* as long as he has not been excommunicated.[66] Even if he is excommunicated and cannot be counted as part of a *minyan,* a sinner is allowed to pray in the synagogue unless the congregants strongly object.[67] The *Mishnah Berurah* cites the *Pri Megadim,* who says that this rule applies only if the sinner is one who sins occasionally out of lust or appetite (*mumar le-te'avon*), but a provocative sinner (*mumar le-hachis*) or one who worships idols or who publicly desecrates the Sabbath is judged like a non-Jew and cannot be counted for a *minyan.*[68]

Rabbi Yechiel Weinberg quotes earlier Hungarian rabbis who say that today no Jew is excommunicated and, therefore, all Jews, even sinners, can be counted as part of a *minyan.*[69] However, he continues, other rabbis say that if a person is worthy of being excommunicated by virtue of transgressions he has committed, he cannot be counted as part of a *minyan* even though he is not actually excommunicated. The clarification of this rabbinic disagreement is important, for homosexuality is a sin for which the transgressor is worthy of being excommunicated. Nevertheless, this responsum of Rabbi Weinberg is difficult to understand in view of the clear statement in *Shulchan Aruch* that unless the sinner is actually excommunicated, he may be counted as part of a *minyan*.

Can Patients with AIDS Lead Synagogue Services?

The question has been raised as to whether or not a patient with AIDS can lead services in the synagogue as a cantor (*shaliach tzibur*) or Torah reader. Jewish law requires that the cantor be worthy, be free of sins, and not have a bad name even when he was younger.[70] Moreover, he should be humble and desired by the congregants, have a sweet voice, and study Torah regularly. Rabbi Moshe Isserles asserts that if someone transgresses unintentionally (*beshogeg*) and repents, he is allowed to serve as a *shaliach tzibur*, but not if he sinned intentionally (*bemayzid*) because he had a bad name before he repented.[71] The *Mishnah Berurah* cites *Magen Avraham*, who quotes many rabbinic decisors that even if one sinned intentionally, he can serve as a *shaliach tzibur* if he repents.[72] However, on fast-days and on the High Holy Days, one should not appoint him as a cantor, although once appointed he should not be removed.

For the High Holy Days, one should seek out a cantor who is most worthy, most learned in Torah, has performed many meritorious deeds, is married, and is over thirty years of age.[73] The *Mishnah Berurah* adds that the cantor and the one who blows the *shofar* should have fully repented from their sins, although one who begins as a cantor or *shofar* blower should not be removed.[74] It thus seems that if an AIDS patient has repented for his sins, including the sin of homosexuality, and if he meets the above qualifications and is acceptable to the congregation, it is permissible to have him lead synagogue services or blow the *shofar* or read from the Torah.

Should a Kohen with AIDS Recite the Priestly Blessing?

Is it permissible for a *kohen* to offer the priestly benediction (go up to the *duchan*) if he has AIDS related to homosexuality or drug addiction? The *Shulchan Aruch* states that if a *kohen* kills someone even unintentionally he should not offer the priestly blessing even if he repents.[75] Ramo adds, in the name of many rabbinic decisors: "If he repents, he is allowed to recite the priestly blessing, and this is the practice which one should follow."

The *Shulchan Aruch* also asserts that if the *kohen* is an apostate he should not recite the priestly blessing, although some rabbis allow him to do so if he repents.[76] If a *kohen* is intoxicated, he should not recite the priestly blessing.[77] So, too, if he married a divorced woman.[78]

However, continues Rav Karo, if none of the above circumstances which prevent a *kohen* from reciting the priestly blessing are present, even if he is not careful about the observance of other commandments, he is allowed to recite the blessing.[79] The *Mishnah Berurah* explains that such commandments include even serious prohibitions such as forbidden sexual relationships (*arayot*).[80] It would appear, therefore, that a *kohen* with AIDS is permitted to offer the priestly benediction. *Mishnah Berurah*, quoting the *Zohar*, adds that if the *kohen* is despised by the congregation, he should not recite the priestly blessing.[81] The reason why even a *kohen* who has sinned is allowed to offer the priestly blessing is that one should not prevent him from performing the positive commandment of blessing the people, thus adding to his sins by not allowing him to fulfill this and other commandments.[82]

Someone might ask: what good is his blessing if he is a sinner? The answer is that the *kohen* only recites the words but the actual blessing comes from G-d, as it is written: *and I will bless them.*[83]

Should a Patient with AIDS Be Honored in the Synagogue?

The Talmud states that it is prohibited to flatter the wicked in this world because it encourages them to believe that they are not doing anything wrong.[84] Furthermore, if a homosexual AIDS patient is honored in the synagogue by being called up to the Torah, people may be misled into thinking that his behavior is acceptable. Thus honoring a sinner might constitute transgression of the negative precept of *not placing a stumbling block before the blind*.[85] The same question arises when a person who publicly violates biblical commandments is honored at a testimonial dinner. Is not the bestowing of such an honor prohibited because it misleads the sinner and the public into believing that the person's violations are being condoned?

Rabbi Feinstein discusses the case of a very philanthropic and charitable Jewish physician who performs many deeds of loving-kindness but is married to a non-Jewish woman.[86] Ordinarily, one should not give this physician any honors in the synagogue because of "the stumbling block that is being placed before the blind" in that such honors might mislead him into believing that his marriage to a non-Jew is not wrong. However, if the honor might lead the sinner to repent, or if one tells him that what he is doing is wrong, it is permissible to give him the honor. In the case under discussion, Rav Feinstein concludes that it is permissible to have the physician open and close the holy ark and remove and subsequently return the Torah to the ark because all the congregants know that he is being honored because of his philanthropy and good deeds, thus the honor does not represent acquiescence to his wrongdoing. Furthermore, the public is in need of his services (*rabim tzerichim loh*) because of his expertise as a physician, and he may, therefore, be accorded the aforementioned honor.

However, the *Chatam Sofer* rules that one should not call a sinner to the Torah for a portion of the Torah reading (*aliyah*) because of the aforementioned possibility of misleading the sinner and/or the public into believing that the sin is being condoned.[87]

Can a Patient with AIDS Serve as a Witness?

Maimonides lists ten classes of individuals who are ineligible to attest or testify before a Jewish court: women, slaves, minors, the mentally deficient, deaf-mutes, the blind, transgressors, the contemptible, relatives, and interested parties.[88] Transgressors are ineligible as witnesses by biblical law, for it is written: *Put not thy hand with the wicked to be an unrighteous witness*,[89] which is interpreted as "accept not the wicked as a witness."[90] Maimonides then enumerates the various types of transgressors, including those who are liable to be flogged, thieves, robbers, tricksters, gamblers, usurers, as well as idlers and vagabonds who are suspected of spending their leisure time in criminal activity.[91]

How should one classify the transgressions of homosexuality and drug addiction, the most common risk factors for the development of AIDS? Those who sin unintentionally are eligible to serve as witnesses, but AIDS patients who are homosexuals know what they are doing. Perhaps such patients can be considered to lack self-control over their strong desire: Jewish law states that a person who sins under compulsion is divinely exempted from punishment (*onus rachamanah patrey*). Support for this position can be found in the talmudic commentary known as *Tosafot*,[92] which quotes the passage stating that one who is suspected of adultery is nevertheless eligible as a witness.[93]

Burial, Funeral Rites, and Mourning for an AIDS Patient

Two cases known to this writer involved AIDS patients who died, where the members of the burial society (*chevra kadisha*) refused to perform the ritual purification of the deceased (*taharah*) because of their fear of contracting AIDS. It is now known that one cannot acquire AIDS by casual contact and their fear was unfounded. However, the problem arises with deceased individuals who had a real contagious disease vis-à-vis the ritual purification for the dead. If the members of the burial society can take precautions such as wearing masks, gloves, and gowns, they should do so. If they cannot or will not do so out of fear, they are not obligated to perform the *taharah* because the latter is only a custom and not a law.[94]

Are the laws of mourning (*avelut*) to be observed for a homosexual patient who died of AIDS? Jewish law states that there is no mourning for those who cast off the yoke of commandments and act like apostates.[95] However, if they repent, mourning is observed for them. Rabbi Abraham Sofer distinguishes between a sinner who suffers for weeks, months, or years before his death and one who dies suddenly. The former probably repented, the latter did not. Therefore, AIDS patients who suffer for variable periods of time before their death should probably be mourned on the assumption that they repented.[96]

It is certainly not proper to honor an AIDS patient after death by naming a school or playground after him. The Talmud interprets the biblical phrase, *But the name of the wicked shall rot*,[97] to mean that rottenness enters their names in that none name their children after them.[98] If it is public knowledge that the AIDS patient was a sinner, he should not be honored after death by having a person or thing named after him. It is also a punishment for the wicked not to honor them after death.

Use of a Mikvah by Women Fearful of Contracting AIDS

The Talmud states that if wine or olive sap falls into a ritual bath or ritualarium (mikvah) and changes its color, it becomes invalid.[99] Based on this ruling, some rabbis prohibit the addition of chlorine to a mikvah because the color of the water is changed to green. As a result of this prohibition, some women are afraid of using such a mikvah for fear of contracting AIDS from the water used by other women whose husbands may have AIDS. However, this fear is totally unfounded, since AIDS cannot be transmitted through water but only by sexual contact or through blood or blood products. Secondly, most rabbis do not prohibit the use of chlorine, because only a minute amount is used to provide antisepsis of the mikvah water. (Sufficient chlorine to make the water change color to green would be intolerable to humans and produce serious eye irritation and skin burning. The greenish color of some mikva'ot is due to the green or blue tiles lining the mikvah.) Furthermore, the rabbis who prohibit the use of chlorine because of the problem of the change in the appearance (*shinuy mareh*) of the water can offer the solution of using chlorine crystals rather than liquid chlorine. The addition of solids such as foods or chemicals, states the talmudic commentary called *Mishnah Acharonah*, does not invalidate a mikvah even if the color of the water is thereby changed.[100]

Circumcision of a Baby with AIDS

The AIDS virus can be transmitted through the placenta from an AIDS-suffering woman, usually a drug addict or sexual partner of an AIDS man, to her unborn fetus. AIDS in newborns or infants is a rare but well-recognized disorder. Is it permissible or mandatory to perform a ritual circumcision (*brit milah*) on such a male infant on the eighth day of life? Must it be postponed until the child recovers from the illness? But there is no cure for AIDS! How does one perform the *metzitzah,* or sucking, which is part of the ritual circumcision? May *metzitzah* be omitted in cases of AIDS?

In a lengthy article, Dr. Abraham Steinberg discusses medical-halachic considerations in the performance of *brit milah.*[101] He reviews the reasons for this divine commandment and the various medical conditions for which the circumcision may or must be postponed. Steinberg cites numerous rabbinic responsa which address these issues. The rules on these matters can be found in the classic codes of Maimonides and Rav Joseph Karo.[102]

If an infant has a generalized illness from which he is not expected to recover, but the physicians state that circumcision would not in any way endanger the infant nor add to the illness, *brit milah* should be performed, preferably on the eighth day.[103] Some rabbis rule that a baby who cannot live for twelve months should be circumcised on a weekday but not on the Sabbath.[104] The *Chatam Sofer* gave a similar ruling in the case of a baby who was not expected to live three months.[105]

On the other hand, Rabbi Bakshi-Doron refused to allow a baby with spina bifida and paraplegia to be circumcised in spite of the medical testimony that the baby had no feeling in the lower half of his body and would not be harmed medically by a *brit milah.*[106] This rabbi and others rule that circumcision should be postponed in any baby with a generalized illness "until it recovers." Most infants with AIDS are critically ill, and circumcision is usually medically and therefore halachically contraindicated.

Conclusion

At the same time that we condemn homosexuality as an immoral act characterized in the Torah as an abomination, we are nevertheless duty bound to defend the basic rights to which homosexuals are entitled. The Torah teaches that even one who is tried, convicted, and executed for a capital crime is still entitled to the respect due to any human being created in the image of G-d. Thus, his corpse may not go unburied overnight.[107] The plight of Jewish AIDS victims doomed to almost certain death should arouse our compassion.

In Judaism, the value of human life is infinite. Whether a person is a homosexual or not, we are obligated to give him proper care if he is sick, charity if he is needy, food if he is hungry, and a burial after death. If he breaks a law of the Torah, he will be punished according to the transgression. Even if AIDS is a punishment by G-d for the sin of homosexuality, Jewish tradition teaches us that such a divine affliction may serve as an atonement for that sin or the patient may repent while ill, making the AIDS victim even more deserving of our mercy and loving-kindness as a fellow Jew.

The compassion of Jewish law in requiring treatment for AIDS patients, however, should not be confused with acquiescence to the behavior of homosexuals who develop AIDS. Under no circumstances does Judaism condone homosexuality, which we characterize as an abomination. Nevertheless, the patient with AIDS should be treated and his life saved. To stand idly by and see the homosexual die without trying to help him is prohibited.[108] Evil should be banned, but the evildoers should be helped to repent.[109]

Notes

1. Leviticus 18:22.
2. Ibid. 20:13.
3. *Sanhedrin* 54a.
4. *Mishneh Torah, Hilchot Issurei Biah* 1:14.
5. I. Jakobovits, *Encyclopaedia Judaica* (Jerusalem: Keter, 1972), vol. 8, cols. 961–962.
6. Genesis 19:5.

7. Judges 19:20.

8. *Sotah* 13b and Jerusalem Talmud, *Sanhedrin* 6:6, 23c.

9. Sanhedrin 57b–58a.

10. "Homosexuality and Judaism," *Journal of Halacha and Contemporary Society* 2 (Spring 1986): 70–87.

11. Responsa *Iggerot Moshe, Yoreh Deah*, vol. 3, no. 35.

12. See F. Rosner, *Modern Medicine and Jewish Ethics*, 2nd rev. ed. (Hoboken, N.J., Ktav, 1991), pp. 391–403.

13. Deuteronomy 4:9.

14. Ibid. 4:15.

15. Ibid. 22:8.

16. *Mishneh Torah, Hilchot Rotze'ach* 11:4 ff.

17. *Shulchan Aruch, Choshen Mishpat* 427 and *Yoreh Deah* 116.

18. *Baba Kamma* 91b.

19. *Mishneh Torah, Hilchot Chovel Umazik* 5:1.

20. *Shulchan Aruch, Choshen Mishpat* 420:31 and *Orach Chayim* 571.

21. Exodus 21:19.

22. *Baba Kamma* 85a.

23. Deuteronomy 22:2.

24. *Mishneh Torah, Hilchot Rotze'ach* 1:14.

25. Rosner, *Modern Medicine and Jewish Ethics*, pp. 7–13.

26. *Shulchan Aruch, Orach Chayim* 328:2.

27. *Sanhedrin* 27b.

28. Ibid. 73a.

29. D. Novak, personal communication. [See below, pp. 000–000. Ed.]

30. *Avodah Zarah* 26b.

31. *Mishneh Torah, Hilchot Rotze'ach* 10:12.

32. Commentary of *Tosafot, Avodah Zarah* 26b, s.v. *ani*; Maimonides' *Mishnah Commentary* on *Nedarim* 4:4; *Shulchan Aruch, Choshen Mishpat* 425:5.

33. *Sanhedrin* 73a; *Shulchan Aruch, Choshen Mishpat* 426:1, *Orach Chayim* 329:8.

34. *Shulchan Aruch, Orach Chayim* 329:8.

35. *Mishnah Berurah* 329:19; *Pitchei Teshuvah, Choshen Mishpat* 426:2.

36. *Mishnah Berurah* 328.

37. Psalms 116:6.

38. *Yebamot* 12b.

39. Responsa *Iggrot Moshe, Even Haezer*, no. 63.

40. *Torat Chesed, Even Haezer*, no. 44; *Achiezer*, part 1, no. 23.

41. Y. L. Zilberstein, *Assia* 11, no. 11 (Nissan 5746–May 1986): 5–11.

42. M. Hershler, *Halacha Urefuah* 2 (1981): 52–57; M. Y. Sloshitz, ibid. 3 (1983): 158–163; A. Metzger, *Harefuah Le'or HaHalachah*, 4 (1985): 10–34; A. S. Abraham, *Hamayan* 22[3] (Nissan 5742), 31–40.

43. A. S. Abraham, *Assia* 5 (1986): 18–23.

44. *Terumot*, end of chap. 8, according to *Ha'amek She'elah, She'iltot* 147:1.

45. Known as *Hagahot Maimuniyot*.

46. *Keseph Mishneh* Commentary of *Hilchot Rotze'ach* 1:14.

47. *Bet Yoseph, Tur Shulchan Aruch, Choshen Mishpat* 426.

48. *Sanhedrin* 73a, according to *Agudat Aizov, Derushim,*. fol. 3b, and *Hashmatot*, fol. 38b.

49. *Radvaz*, pt. 5 (p. 2 in *Leshonot HaRambam*, sec. 1, 582); *Radvaz*, pt. 3, no. 627, and *Sheiltot Radvaz* 1:52.

50. Leviticus 19:16.

51. Responsa *Iggrot Moshe, Yoreh Deah*, pt. 2. no. 174:4; Responsa *Tzitz Eliezer*, vol. 10, no. 25:7.

52. O. Yosef, *Halachah Urefuah* 3 (1983): 61–63; J. J. Weiss, Responsa *Minchat Yitzchok*, pt. 6, no. 103:2; Responsa *Tzitz Eliezer*, vol. 10, no. 25:7. See also M. Meiselman, *Halachah Urefuah* 2 (1981): 114–121; M. Hershler, ibid. 2 (1981): 122–127.

53. Genesis 18:1.

54. *Sotah* 14a.

55. I. Jakobovits, *Journal of a Rabbi* (New York: Living Books, 1966), p. 156.

56. Responsa *Ramo*, no. 9 (end).

57. *Nedarim* 39b, *Berachot* 22b, and *Rashi* on *Shabbat* 30a.

58. I. Jakobovits, *Jewish Medical Ethics* (New York: Bloch, 1959), pp. 108–109.

59. J. Cassuto, *Jahrbuch der Juedisch-Literarischen Gesellschaft* 10 (1912): 252 and 280 (in minutes dated 1664 and 1666).

60. J. J. Greenwald. *Kol Bo Al Avelut* (New York/Jerusalem, Feldheim, 1947–51), p. 17.

61. *Mishneh Torah, Hilchot Shemirat Hanefesh* 1:7.

62. *Pesachim* 8b.

63. *Turei Zahav (Taz)* on *Shulchan Aruch, Orach Chayim* 455:3.

64. Sanhedrin 73a.

65. Rosner, *Modern Medicine and Jewish Ethics*, pp. 375–390.

66. *Shulchan Aruch, Orach Chayim* 55:11.

67. Ibid. 55:12.

68. *Mishnah Berurah* 55:11:46.

69. Responsa *Seridei Aish*, pt. 2, no. 6.

70. *Shulchan Aruch, Orach Chayim* 53:4.

71. *Ramo* on *Orach Chayim* 53:5.

72. *Mishnah Berurah* 53:5:22.

73. *Ramo* on *Orach Chayim* 581:1.

74. *Mishnah Berurah* 581:1:11.

75. *Shulchan Aruch, Orach Chayim* 128:35.

76. Ibid. 128:37.

77. Ibid. 128:38.

78. Ibid. 128:40.

79. Ibid. 128:39.

80. *Mishnah Berurah* 128:39:143.

81. Ibid. 128:10:37.

82. *Hasagot of Ramah* (Jerusalem, 5744/1984), *Hilchot Nesiyat Kapayim* 18:6.
83. Numbers 6:27.
84. Sotah 41b.
85. Leviticus 19:14.
86. Responsa *Iggrot Moshe, Orach Chayim,* pt. 2, no. 51.
87. Responsa *Chatam Sofer, Orach Chayim,* no. 15.
88. *Mishneh Torah, Hilchot Eydut* 9:1.
89. Exodus 23:1.
90. *Mishneh Torah, Hilchot Eydut* 10:1.
91. Ibid. 10:2–5.
92. *Tosafot* on Sanhedrin 9b, s.v. *liretzono.*
93. *Sanhedrin* 26b.
94. *Chochmat Adam,* beginning of the customs of the *chevra kadisha.*
95. *Shulchan Aruch, Yoreh Deah* 345:5.
96. Responsa *Ketav Sofer, Yoreh Deah,* no. 171.
97. Proverbs 10:7.
98. *Yoma* 38b.
99. *Mikva'ot* 7:3.
100. Ibid.
101. A. Steinberg, *Assia* (5743/1983): 207–228.
102. *Mishneh Torah, Hilchot Milah* 1:1 ff.; *Shulchan Aruch, Yoreh Deah* 260 ff.
103. Responsa *Minchat Yitzchok,* vol. 5, no. 11.
104. Responsa *Maharam Schick, Yoreh Deah,* no. 243.
105. Responsa *Chatam Sofer,* no. 64.
106. E. Bakshi-Doron, *Halachah Urefuah* 2 (1981): 268–272.
107. Deuteronomy 21:23.
108. Leviticus 19:16.
109. Psalms 104:35.

AIDS: Jewish Perspectives (1990)

ל״ב

Abraham Steinberg

Introduction

Several important facts constitute the basis for the ethical impact of the acquired immunodeficiency syndrome (AIDS): the disease is fatal, communicable, stigmatizing, and expensive to treat.

The prospects for a vaccine or a cure are unfortunately at least several years away. The median survival period of AIDS patients from time of diagnosis is about one year. No patient clinically ill with AIDS has survived the disease.

AIDS is an expensive disease to treat. Total lifetime hospitalization cost per AIDS patient in the United States is estimated to be from $80,000 to $147,000.[1] In addition to direct medical costs, AIDS places a tremendous burden on public health services, including hospital beds, acute- and chronic-care facilities, and personnel resources. AIDS also causes an enormous loss of potential earnings due to disability from the disease itself and premature death of young persons, who comprise the great majority of the disease's victims. The income lost per patient in the United States is estimated to be about $490,000.[2]

The AIDS crisis has brought many ethical issues to the forefront with great intensity. None of these moral concerns, however, is unique to AIDS: the patient-physician relationship, confidentiality, informed consent, truth telling, attitude to the dying person, "life-support" systems, experimental therapies, allocation of scarce resources, screening and quarantine policies—all are part and parcel of medical ethics at large. This chapter deals with some of these issues.

AIDS is not the first communicable, incurable, fatal disease that has challenged the human race.[3] Societies responded to plagues and sexual diseases in previous times with fear similar to that we are currently experiencing with AIDS. In the mid-fourteenth century, the Black Death pandemic traveled from Asia into Europe and caused the death of many people.[4] For over a century, as doctors battled smallpox, yellow fever, leprosy, typhoid, tuberculosis, gonorrhea, and syphilis, American courts struggled to balance society's interest in protecting the public by controlling communicable diseases, particularly sexually transmitted diseases, versus the individual's claim to constitutional liberty.[5] Even today, many other disorders such as malignancies, cardiovascular diseases, neurodegenerative disorders, and severe malformations are incurable, cause severe pain and suffering, and occur in much greater numbers than AIDS. Yet these disorders do not cause the same amount of alarm and concern as does AIDS.

Nonetheless, AIDS involves special and distinctive ethical issues in the aggregate, since it poses many varied problems of great intensity, all related to a single disease. AIDS is also a stigmatizing disease, since it is often related to homosexuality or drug addiction. The dislike of homosexuals—homophobia—is quite common. In one survey, a small but significant minority of AIDS care givers felt that their homosexual patients with AIDS were "getting what they deserve."[6] The other large group of AIDS patients—drug addicts—is notoriously unpopular on hospital wards. Some care givers and others opine that AIDS in drug addicts is self-inflicted, thereby giving them less right to proper care.

There may, however, be other sociocultural reasons for the worldwide concern about the AIDS epidemic. AIDS affects an affluent society that is highly self-confident, where science and technology have known practically no bounds to success in the prevention and cure of communicable diseases. Many people believe that infectious diseases in the late twentieth century were confined to underdeveloped countries or readily controlled by modern therapy. AIDS does not fit this blueprint. How, then, should society approach this mysterious and ultimately fatal disease in an era of such high technology? How can a prosperous society cope with this catastrophe? A resident physician who trained in New York City, most of whose patients were afflicted with AIDS, concluded:

> We alone, of all our peers and all our successors, have had during our training a brief glimpse of medicine as it used to be. We learned to practice clinical medicine as it was before the age of technology. . . . For five years we grew accustomed to watching our AIDS patients die amid all the glitter of medical technology, while we could offer them only comfort, sympathy, and palliation. . . . Still, a few of us have had a powerful lesson in history and humility, which can only serve us well in the complicated days ahead.[7]

AIDS also affects primarily young people, thus creating more emotional concern compared with other terminal conditions affecting mostly old people. Further, AIDS initially involved many celebrities of the media and the entertainment world whose plight was widely publicized.

These negative reflections, however, are not aimed at discouraging strong efforts to control, prevent, and cure this illness. They merely point out some of the psychosocial elements involved in the panic surrounding the disease.

Ethical Dilemmas Involving the Care of AIDS Patients

The goals of any proposed policy regarding AIDS should be clear and uncontroversial: (a) to help individual victims by alleviating pain, anguish, and suffering, and by striving for an eventual cure; and (b) to safeguard the health of the public by minimizing and eventually eliminating the spread of the disease. The problem is how to achieve these goals. In the United States, until 1989, more than 170 laws and regulations concerning AIDS were enacted, and courts and human rights commission decisions were issued.[8] These laws pertain to prevention, education, screening, reporting, and antidiscrimination. In spite of these laws, many difficult ethical problems still remain to be broached before an optimal solution is reached. Indeed, several hundred publications pertaining to AIDS and ethics have been published to date.[9]

"Moral Etiology" of AIDS

Some people place the blame for the AIDS epidemic directly on the promiscuous life-style of high-risk-group patients. The affliction of AIDS is regarded as a straightforward punishment for sinful behavior. Some people have even voiced the opinion that AIDS victims have no "right" to expensive health care facilities, because they brought the disease upon themselves by immoral or illicit behavior. This approach is morally unacceptable, since a direct cause-and-effect relationship between sinful life and AIDS cannot and should not be ascribed by ordinary people, and should not be involved when treatment and compassion are decisions to be made.

In Judaism, God cherishes the life of every human being. The preservation of human life takes precedence over almost all religious commandments. Every life is worth saving, without distinction as to whether the person whose life is in danger is a criminal, transgressor, or law-abiding citizen.[10] King Solomon taught us that there is not a just man upon earth that does good and sins not,[11] and the talmudic sages taught us that there is no death without sin.[12] Thus, everyone is guilty of at least some sins. Therefore, physicians and other health-care providers should not act as judges; they are obliged to heal and care for all patients, including AIDS victims. Whether or not a person is a homosexual, a drug addict, attempts suicide, or desecrates the Sabbath, one is obligated to render him proper care if he is sick. Evil should be banned, but evildoers should be helped to repent.[13] Therefore, patients with AIDS, particularly those who are driven, perhaps subconsciously, to their sinful activities out of lust and bad habits, should be treated no differently from other patients.

Prevention of AIDS

There is as yet no cure for AIDS. Therefore, effective preventive measures are vital. Education is currently the major weapon against the spread of AIDS. Education involves both those who are infected and those who are not. The content of the educational campaign, however, is ethically charged and requires further analysis.

Since the social philosophy of current Western society is heavily based upon the principle of autonomy, and since our society has accepted homosexuality as an alternative life-style, the current content of the educational campaign has a flavor that does not correspond with an authentic Jewish approach.

The mode of HIV transmission is well established: it occurs only through sexual contact, contact with infected needles, the administration of infected blood or blood products, and placental transfer from mother to fetus. One way of reducing the transmissibility of the virus is by eliminating its spread through sexual contact. Government officials, professionals of all kinds, and particularly the media, strongly advocate sex education recommending the use of condoms, which are identified as "lifeguards." An editorial in the *American Journal of Medicine* by Emanuel and Emanuel in 1987 seriously questioned the ethics of this campaign for "safe sex" and concluded:

> The message of the current "safe sex" campaign is untrue and therefore unethical. . . . Further, those individuals who do heed the public health warnings are lulled into a false sense of security. . . . Furthermore, the "safe sex" campaign may also be counter-productive. . . . If people are led to believe that condoms eliminate HIV transmission, they may not reduce the frequency of sexual relations. . . . it is ethically impermissible to use distorted slogans, partial information, and exaggerated claims; we can not offer people false security in the hope of persuading them to act more prudently.[14]

From the Jewish point of view, this educational campaign is morally wrong. The Bible labels homosexuality as an abomination and ordains capital punishment for both transgressors.[15] Homosexuality is strictly banned in Jewish law, the prohibition being applied to both Jews and non-Jews.[16] It is viewed as an unnatural perversion debasing the dignity of man, frustrating the procreative purpose of sex, and damaging family life. Jewish law rejects the view that homosexuality is merely a disease or morally neutral, and Judaism certainly does not accept the interpretation of an "alternative sexual preference."[17] The homosexual act is regarded as a grave sin, and despite tendencies and urges to commit this sin, it is required that a human being struggle against these inclinations as much as he is able, no different than grappling with tendencies to murder or to steal. If the sin was committed under coercive internal forces, the court may consider that fact when punishment is discussed, but an individual is not exempt from fighting his evil tendencies. Ideological homosexuality is most reprehensible in the Jewish view and should be strongly discouraged via educational methods.

Western society has become increasingly hedonistic, with a sexual revolution characterized by a steady deterioration in sex inhibitions and by increasing permissiveness. These current attitudes are profoundly at variance with traditional Jewish views on sex and sexual morality.

The Jewish view on homosexuality is not a popular one; however, it seems more correct today than ever before, taking into account the high risks involved in such behavior. AIDS, as well as other serious infectious diseases such as syphilis, gonorrhea, hepatitis, and herpes, is much more prevalent among homosexuals. These facts should be sufficient reason to demand a change in the life-style of homosexuals. Thus the current campaign that promotes the use of condoms but fully legitimizes homosexuality is morally wrong. An additional halachic issue is the violation of improper emission of semen due to the use of a condom.[18]

The other major risk group consists of drug addicts. Drug abuse is also a forbidden act in Jewish law. Drug addiction is prohibited because it endangers life and health, and the Torah instructs us not to intentionally place ourselves in danger: "Take heed to thyself, and take care of thy life."[19] Hence the abuse of intravenous narcotics, which constitutes a definite danger and hazard to life, is considered a pernicious habit and is thus prohibited.[20] Drug addiction also increases the crime rate and severely affects personal competency and responsibility.

The ethical dilemma of the constitutional balance between the preservation of the public health and liberty for the individual is a long and changing endeavor in human moral and legal debates. In the United States, courts at the turn of the twentieth century strongly endorsed the power of the states to adopt stringent measures controlling contagious diseases, provided these measures were reasonable. Courts at that time frequently noted that medical experts, not judges, should decide technical questions.[21] In recent years the courts' rulings in the United States have markedly changed. The view that individual rights represent independent, positive weights of different values has become firmly entrenched in constitutional decision making. The courts are balancing the public health risks against individual rights, and are of the opinion that civil liberties need not invariably yield to the public health.[22]

Most forces in current Western societies, however, have found the balance between public health and individual liberty difficult to strike, and no lasting balance has yet been achieved. Moralists in general believe that certain forms of behavior must be observed if society's central orders—religion, work, family, and relations between the sexes—are to be upheld. All laws are repressive to some extent. Morality is concerned with the change of human behavior and the striving for improving man and society. The balance of societal needs versus individual liberties makes the difference between anarchy, totalitarianism, and democracy.

Lord Patrick Devlin criticized a British committee's 1957 recommendation to remove criminal sanctions for private homosexual conduct. He wrote: "What makes a society of any sort is a community of ideas, not only political ideas, but also ideas about the way its members should behave and govern their lives. . . . Without shared ideas on politics, morals and ethics no society can exist."[23]

In Judaism, explicit halachic rulings invalidate the notion of autonomy; therefore, one cannot use the principle of self-determination or the right of privacy to commit an act that is forbidden according to halachah, even when there is no harm to others. The autonomy of man, in Jewish ethics, is restricted to conduct that is in accordance with the law. Autonomy is completely waived when it leads to harm, destruction, and violation of life and health, whether one's own or that of others. Respect for persons and their self-determination is rightfully due only to those who have self-respect for the preservation of life.[24]

Therefore, sexual practices that threaten public health are not beyond the reach of public regulations, providing their ill effects are soundly proven. Homosexuality can no longer be considered an innocent private mode of sexual practice, since statistical data prove that it is a serious health hazard.[25] Jewish law, which prohibits homosexual conduct, serves as a vital barrier against AIDS. If homosexuality were to decline sharply, the number of AIDS cases would, in turn, decrease. Similarly, Judaism would oppose the distribution of sterile needles to intravenous drug users as a strategy to stop the spread of AIDS, since drug use is not just a health problem, it is a vice.

A genuine educational campaign, therefore, should stress the wrongfulness of the behavior of homosexuals and drug addicts. These life-styles have led to serious health problems for the involved individuals as well as to society. The educational campaign, therefore, should emphasize the importance of avoiding such behavior patterns. Legislation banning these acts should be enacted. These acts should not be legitimized or encouraged by campaigns for "safe sex" and disposable needles. Since drug addiction is becoming the major risk factor for AIDS in Western society and education for drug addicts has only limited success, society has a moral obligation to establish more and better drug addiction preventive and treatment programs, as well as better law-enforcement measures against dealers, distributors, and drug users.

Moral Obligations of Health-Care Providers to Treat AIDS Patients

Is a physician or other health-care provider ethically obliged to care for a patient with AIDS, or is he morally justified in refraining from caring for him, for fear of contracting the disease? What are the objective data concerning the risks of health-care givers becoming infected by the AIDS virus? Physicians have been reported to be reluctant to care for patients with AIDS primarily because of fear of infection with HIV.[26] Anesthetists have been reluctant to give anesthetics, surgeons to perform lung biopsies, pathologists to handle specimens or do autopsies, and dentists to treat seropositive patients.[27] Clinicians at large were found to be ignorant of the true meaning of HIV infection, hence behaving in an inappropriate manner toward such patients.[28] Not only doctors, but also nurses, social workers, and ambulance drivers have voiced serious concern about treating AIDS patients.[29] Caring for the sick has always been a somewhat hazardous occupation. Medical personnel taking care of patients with typhus, tuberculosis, or hepatitis B knew they risked infection that could even be fatal.

The facts concerning AIDS, however, are different. It is not inherently unsafe for healthy people to care for AIDS patients, because the virus is transmitted only through the exchange of blood or semen. There is no evidence of the disease having been transmitted by casual contact or during the health care of AIDS patients, unless there is parenteral inoculation or exchange of body fluids through nonintact skin or mucosa.[30] Thus AIDS patients and HIV carriers do not represent a substantial risk for doctors.[31] In Judaism, healing the sick is a positive commandment, not simply a trade for the purpose of earning income. Therefore, the physician should be prepared for inconveniences and remote complications, as defined in and qualified by halachah.

The question as to whether or not a person is obligated, according to Jewish law, to subject himself to a risk in order to save another person's life is discussed in great detail in rabbinic sources. Halachah requires that one help, save, or heal any fellowman. Based on the biblical verse: "Thou shalt not stand against the blood of thy neighbor,"[32] the Talmud states that if one sees his neighbor drowning or mauled by beasts or attacked by robbers, he is bound to save him.[33] However, if there is danger involved to the rescuer, it would depend on the calculated risk involved. The prevailing opinion seems to be the following, based on a responsum by the *Radbaz:* If there is great danger to the rescuer, he is not allowed to attempt to save his fellowman. If the danger to the rescuer is small and the danger to his fellowman is great, the rescuer is allowed but not obligated to attempt the rescue. If there is no risk at all to the rescuer, or if the risk is very small or remote, he is obligated to try to save his fellow-man. If he refuses to do so, he is guilty of transgressing the above-mentioned biblical commandment. Since the risk to health personnel in caring for AIDS patients is very small, certainly less than the risk involved in saving a person attacked by robbers, it follows that the physician is obligated under Jewish law to care for such patients.[34]

Not only is a physician obliged to treat AIDS patients, but there is also the duty incumbent upon everyone to visit the sick. This act is considered to be a highly benevolent act, and since the risk of contracting AIDS by visiting or touching the AIDS patient appears to be nil, the commandment to visit the sick is applicable in this disease as well.[35]

Confidentiality and Coercive Screening

The requirement of confidentiality is to keep the patient's information entrusted by him to the physician. This requirement is based upon moral as well as practical considerations. According to halachah, this requirement is included in the prohibition of rechilut (talebearing) and lashon hara (speaking evil). However, an ethical and halachic dilemma arises in cases where keeping the secrets of the patient may cause harm to a third innocent party. In such circumstances, halachah clearly requires the prevention of damage to others, and the prohibition of rechilut does not apply. This ruling is limited by certain provisions. First of all, one should make an effort to convince the patient to share his secret with potentially endangered persons. When such efforts fail, one should disclose the information only to the potentially affected persons, and only when one is absolutely certain about the facts.[36] Thus, if the physician of record knows that a patient suffers from AIDS, it is his obligation to verify the diagnosis and let the patient's sexual partners know about it. This approach is also accepted by the American Medical Association's House of Delegates.[37]

In Jewish law, the obligation to protect the life and health of the public takes precedence over personal autonomy and the right of privacy. Therefore, if mass screening for HIV can be beneficial to minimize the spread of AIDS, there is no halachic hindrance to applying even coercive screening.[38] However, public health policy experts state that such methods are not beneficial in reaching the goal of better controlling the spread of AIDS, and therefore coercive screening should not be used.[39]

Several other ethical issues are of paramount importance and deserve an in-depth comparative moral assessment. These include the issues of truth telling, attitude to the dying patient, experimental therapies, and allocation of scarce resources, among others. These and other issues have to be seriously debated, and an optimal balance must be achieved between conflicting ethical dilemmas. These debates should be based primarily on scientifically sound data and followed by halachic decisions as interpreted and applied only by qualified rabbinic decisors.

Conclusion

In order to keep intact the fabric of a pluralistic, democratic society while facing the enormous ethical burden posed by the AIDS catastrophe, it is mandatory to evaluate and debate frankly and honestly all aspects from all points of view. An optimal balance must be achieved between the conflicting ethical dilemmas. The solution from the Jewish point of view must be reached through scientifically and halachically sound bases, as interpreted by the authoritative decisors.

Notes

1. D. E. Bloom and G. Carliner, "The Economic Impact of AIDS in the United States," *Science* 239 (1988): 604–610.

2. Ibid.

3. A. Zuger and S. H. Miles, "Physicians, AIDS, and Occupational Risk—Historic Traditions and Ethical Allegations," *JAMA* 258 (1987): 1924–28.

4. R. S. Gottfried, *The Black Death* (New York: Free Press, 1983).

5. D. J. Merritt, "The Constitutional Balance Between Health and Liberty," *Hastings Center Report* 16, no. 6 (1986): S2–S1O; Board of Trustees, American Medical Association, "Prevention and Control of AIDS," *JAMA* 258 (1987): 2097–2103.

6. T. P. Kalman, C. M. Kalman, and C. J. Ougles, "Homophobia Among Physicians and Nurses," Abstract 225, 2nd International Conference on AIDS, Paris, France, June 23–25, 1986.

7.   A. Zuger, "Professional Responsibilities in the AIDS Generation," *Hastings Center Report* 17, no. 3 (1987): 16–20.

8.   L. Gostin, "The AIDS Litigation Project," *JAMA* 263 (1990): 1961–90.

9.   C. Manuel, P. Enal, J. Charrel, et al., "The Ethical Approach to AIDS: A Bibliographical Review," *Journal of Medical Ethics* 16 (1990): 14–27.

10.   *Sanhedrin* 73a.

11.   Ecclesiastes 7:20.

12.   *Shabbat* 55a.

13.   Psalm 104:35, *Berachot* 10a.

14.   E. J. Emanuel and L. L. Emanuel, "Is Our AIDS Policy Ethical?" *American Journal of Medicine* 83 (1987): 519–520.

15.   Leviticus 18:22, 20:13.

16.   Maimonides' *Mishneh Torah, Issure Biah* 1:14, *Melachim* 9:5–6.

17.   I. Jakobovits, "Homosexuality," *Encyclopaedia Judaica* 8 (1972): 961–962; N. Lamm, "Judaism and the Modern Attitude to Homosexuality," *Encyclopaedia Judaica Year Book* (1974), pp. 194–205.

18.   *Responsa Maharsham*, pt. 3, no. 268.

19.   Deuteronomy 4:9. .

20.   M. Feinstein, *Responsa Iggrot Moshe, Yoreh De'ah*, pt. 3, no. 35.

21.   P. Devlin, *The Enforcement of Morals* (Oxford: Oxford University Press, 1959; 1968).

22.   Mezzit, "The Constitutional Balance," (n. 5).

23.   Devlin, *The Enforcement of Morals*.

24.   A. Steinberg, *Encyclopedia Refu'it Hilchatit*, 2nd ed. (1988), vol. 1, pp. 70–74.

25.   Centers for Disease Control, "Update: Acquired Immunodeficiency Syndrome—United States, 1989," *JAMA* 263 (1990): 1191–92.

26.   Health and Public Policy Committee, American College of Physicians, "AIDS," *Annual of Internal Medicine* 104 (1986): 575–581.

27.   E. S. Searle, "Knowledge, Attitudes, and Behavior of Health Professionals in Relation to AIDS," *Lancet* 1 (1987): 26–28.

28.   Ibid.

29.   Ibid.

30.   G. H. Friedland and R. S. Klein, "Transmission of the Human Immunodeficiency Virus," *New England Journal of Medicine* 317 (1987): 1125–35; Searle, "Knowledge, Attitudes."

31.   D. Smith, "AIDS: A Doctor's Duty," *British Medical Journal* 294 (1987): 6.

32.   Leviticus 19:16.

33.   *Sanhedrin* 73a.

34.   *Responsa Radvaz*, vol. 3, no. 627.

35.   A. Steinberg, *Encyclopedia Refu'it Hilchatit*, 2nd ed. (1988), vol. 1, p. 89.

36.   Chafetz Chaim, *Hilchot Issurei Rechilut*, sec. 9.

37.   *New York Times*, June 30, 1989.

38.   Rabbi S. Deichowsky, *Assia,* nos. 45–46 (1989): 28–33. (In this volume, below, pp. 105–112.)

39.   J. Osborn, "AIDS, Politics, and Science," *New England Journal of Medicine* 318 (1988): 444–447.

The Problem of AIDS in a Jewish Perspective (1992)

אבג

David Novak

Current Public Concern with AIDS

Since the discovery, about ten years ago, of the growing health problem of acquired immune deficiency syndrome (AIDS), public concern with this new phenomenon has increased significantly. In fact, public discussion of it has far out-stripped discussion of any other health problem in our society. The media are constantly filled with everything from personal testimonies by and about AIDS sufferers and their loved ones to predictions by various experts on the future course of the prob-lem and how we might best cope with it. Indeed, interest in the problem is so widespread, and fear about it so rampant, that the surgeon general of the United States prepared a booklet about AIDS and how to avoid contracting it. The booklet was sent to every American household.

If AIDS were just a health problem per se, that is, simply a physical disease (actually, it is the result of a virus that weakens the natural immune system of the body to such an extent that there is no effective defense against any infection that might attack the body), the degree of public concern we have seen heretofore might well be out of proportion to the actual physical danger at hand. Despite the growing number of patients dying

73

as the result of AIDS-related diseases, their number is smaller than the number of patients who die as the result of cancer, heart disease, and other more familiar fatal maladies. Moreover, despite warnings by some experts—warnings disputed by other experts—that the general population is at an increasing risk, male homosexuals and intravenous drug users are still the highest-risk groups.[1] Therefore, there must be something about this malady that inspires more than just the fear of imminent physical contagion in the general population, the overwhelming number of whom do not fall into the two highest-risk groups just noted. For most of us, then, AIDS has created more of a spiritual problem, in truth, than a physical one. As such, any human approach to this problem—certainly any religious approach, which must deal with concerns of both body and soul—will be inadequate if it deals with the AIDS problem only as it would with any other epidemic or threatened epidemic. Indeed, it seems that the very phenomenology of AIDS involves religious questions in a more immediate way than any other modern health problem. And because so much of the population has been so thoroughly secularized, certainly in terms of attitudes toward health and disease, the especially religious phenomenology of AIDS is something for which they have been ill prepared by our culture.

The religious phenomenology of AIDS becomes evident in three spiritual issues AIDS inevitably raises. First, AIDS seems to question the prevailing hedonism of our culture, for before the appearance of AIDS, it was far easier to argue that our bodies are simply there to be used for our pleasure, that there are no bodily impediments per se, that we can do with our bodies whatever we will. The availability of antibiotic drugs (that have supposedly cured the old venereal diseases like syphilis and gonorrhea), birth control drugs and devices, and legalized hygienic abortion certainly had made the arguments for a "sexual revolution" more compelling, although the dangers of the drug aspect of this overall *hedonistic revolution* were becoming increasingly evident even before AIDS came on the scene. But AIDS has now demonstrated that the promiscuity that generally characterizes those at greatest risk of contracting it (including more and more heterosexuals) is physically dangerous. In other words, the old warnings about the physical consequences of hedonistic promiscuity ("You'll get a terrible disease if you do that!") suddenly have a new truth about them. AIDS has now shown us that the body is not just the tool of the soul's willful capacity but that it has an inherent integrity of its own that must be respected for the sake of the good of the whole human person. And it has shown that the human will is only part of a larger created nature and that the will's pretensions to omnipotence, pretensions supremely manifest in hedonism, are mortally dangerous on the most immediate physical level.[2] Furthermore, it is important to add, at this point, that our lack of preparation for the AIDS crisis because of our hedonism is in essence akin to our lack of preparation for the whole ecological crisis because of our uncritical faith in technology.[3] In both cases, human pretensions of omnipotence are being directly challenged by the biological order of nature, which is beyond our control.

Second, AIDS seems to raise what was thought by most moderns to be an ancient superstition long behind us, namely, the whole issue of God's punishment of sin through physical maladies. Yet, as anyone with either therapeutic or pastoral experience well knows, the first question most often raised even today, even by many "nonreligious" people, who have discovered serious disease in themselves is: "What did I do for God to do this to me?."[4] Now, in the case of most other diseases, whose epidemiology is totally external, one can attempt to reason with the patient by showing that the disease was contracted through no fault of his or her own. (Whether such "reasoning" is psychologically helpful to this type of patient is another question in and of itself.) Nevertheless, in regard to AIDS, the patient most often does indeed know just what he or she did that caused his or her body to be so receptive to the AIDS virus and thereby set in motion the deadly syndrome.

This entails considerable guilt, for most of the people in our culture, however otherwise secularized they may be, still regard homosexual acts and the use of narcotic drugs to be not only immoral but sinful, that is, they are acts for which God will punish us. Therefore, the cultural message about AIDS seems to be that it is caused not only by one's own acts but by one's immoral or sinful acts. Indeed, one need no longer argue for the immorality of these acts based on abstract philosophical or theological definitions; rather, one can now actually point to concrete and seemingly inevitable consequences. Arguments on behalf of AIDS sufferers that ignore these indisputable facts can be regarded only as rationalizations motivated by pathological denials of empirical reality.

Finally, the fact that children can be born with AIDS because of the acts of their parents seems to raise the old fear that "God punishes the children for the sins of the parents."[5] This fear also applies to those who have contracted AIDS because of having been infused in one way or another with the bodily fluids of someone who did contact AIDS because of his or her own acts. In other words, we suffer not only for our own sins but for the sins of others before us. This raises the whole question of "original sin," a doctrine most Jews (at least most liberal Jews) are surprised if not shocked to learn that Judaism affirms as does Christianity after it, albeit with some important differences.[6]

It is because of these considerations that a Jewish approach to the problem of AIDS must incorporate both the immediately practical norms of Halakhah and, also, some of the more theoretical reflections of Jewish theology about disease in general, reflections that can be seen as informing the whole normative process of which Halakhah is always the most evident aspect.[7] For an adequate Jewish discussion of AIDS must address not only the bodily needs of those specifically afflicted with it but their spiritual needs and, indeed, the spiritual needs of all those for whom the very social presence of AIDS has raised some old religious questions in some surprisingly new ways.

Indiscriminate Treatment of the Sick

It must be emphasized at the very outset that for Traditional Judaism, male homosexual acts are absolutely prohibited, both for Jews and non-Jews. (Female homosexual acts are also prohibited, but their prohibition is based on quite different sources. Moreover, because female homosexuals are not a high-risk AIDS group, we need not be concerned with them in this specific context.)[8] According to one major authority in the Talmud, both Jewish and non-Jewish males are proscribed from homosexual acts by the scriptural prohibition "You shall not lie with a man as with a woman; it is an abomination [*to'evah hi*]" (Leviticus 18:22).[9] According to another authority, this verse specifically proscribes Jewish men only, non-Jewish men being so proscribed by the scriptural verse "a man . . . shall cleave to his wife [and they shall be one flesh]" (Genesis 2:24), which is interpreted to mean "but not with a male [*zakhar*]."[10] This latter interpretation, which is taken to be the normative one, entails the view that the Jewish proscription of such homosexual acts is a reaffirmation of a more general human proscription, whereas the former interpretation sees the Jewish proscription as being primary and the general human proscription as being derivative. The acceptance of this latter interpretation is important in emphasizing that for subsequent Jewish tradition, the proscription of male homosexual acts is neither something applying only to Jews nor something "Jewish" to be imposed on the general population by Jews or by the influence of Judaism. It can be addressed as a human issue per se. Therefore, Traditional Judaism can make common cause with other religious and ethical traditions that affirm the same human proscriptions, without any one of them subordinating its own moral authority to the other.[11]

The same type of moral presentation can be seen in the prohibition of acts that are clearly destructive of life and health, of which intravenous drug use is such an obvious example to everyone by now. Thus one of the main grounds given in the Talmud for this prohibition is the verse addressed to Noah and his sons (for the Rabbis, "sons of Noah" is a synonym for humankind per se), "Surely I shall hold you responsible for your own lifeblood" (Genesis 9:5).[12] Indeed, in a famous passage in the Talmud, where a rabbi being martyred is urged to shorten his suffering by hastening his own death while being burned at the stake, the rabbi refuses, arguing along general human lines that "it is best that He who gave life take it, but that a person not destroy himself."[13]

So we can now see that the majority of AIDS sufferers are considered to be in the category of sinners (including promiscuous
heterosexuals), and it is irrelevant whether they be Jews or non-
Jews. However, this should in no wise prevent full care being
extended to AIDS patients, even though sympathy with their
plight must never lead to approval for their way of life. This
needs to be emphasized because I strongly suspect that there is a
concerted attempt on the part of apologists for homosexuality
(as well as for sexual license of any kind) to extend normal
human sympathy for AIDS suffering in particular to a more general human sympathy for *everything* about those suffering from
AIDS. In terms of Jewish teaching as well as ordinary human
reason, such an extension of sympathy is totally misplaced. It is
as misplaced as attempting to extend our normal human sympathy with smokers suffering from lung cancer to their practice of
smoking cigarettes. Nevertheless, our obligation *to* AIDS
patients must be internalized as sympathy *with* them for three
reasons.

First, according to Jewish tradition, everyone is essentially a
sinner. "There is no person [*adam*] on earth who is so righteous
that he will do only good and not sin" (Ecclesiastes 7:20).[14] And
even certain extraordinary scriptural personalities, who are seen
by the Talmud as being themselves without sin, are still
included in the mortality decreed for all humankind because of
original sin.[15]

Second, the Talmud sees all human suffering as a means for
intensifying our relationship with God. This turns out to mean
that even if a person cannot discern specific sin in oneself when
suffering, one is to act as if he or she were a sinner, namely, he or
she must return to God (the Hebrew for "repentance" is *teshuvah*—"return").[16] Therefore, sin is so pervasively human that the
difference between the righteous and the wicked is ultimately
one of degree, not of kind. This does not, of course, excuse anyone's particular sin, but it does indicate that the self-righteous
confidence that assumes its own security because it is not suffering at present as is someone else, that such self-righteous confidence is religiously abhorrent. As the atonement liturgy used on
Yom Kippur succinctly puts it, "We are neither so arrogant nor

so stubborn as to say before You, O Lord our God and God of our ancestors, that we are righteous [*tsadiqim anahnu*] and have not sinned."[17]

Third, because we are all, therefore, subject to both disease and death due to our sins, we are in an existential position to *sympathize* with (literally "feel with," from the Greek *sympathein*, as in the German *Mitgefuehl*) those suffering from any disease, including AIDS. This is brought out in the rabbinic treatment of the scriptural norms concerning the disease *tsara'at* (wrongly translated "leprosy"; actually a far less fatal disease than what is for us *leprosy*, namely, Hansen's disease). According to the Rabbis, the reason that Scripture specifically singles out this disease for its concern is because it is the punishment for a number of antisocial vices, most especially slander.[18] The community is commanded to quarantine those suffering from this disease.[19] Now it seems that this is for the sake of the community, that it not become contaminated by contact with them, either physically or spiritually. "And the one who is afflicted with the disease [*ve-ha-tsarua*], his clothes shall be rent and his head disheveled, and he shall cover his upper lip and cry 'Unclean! Unclean! [*tame*]'" (Leviticus 13:45). However, the Rabbis emphasize that this is not done to humiliate the *tsara'at* sufferers but to give them the public opportunity to express their pain and anguish and to beseech others to "seek compassion [*rahamim*] for them."[20] *Compassion* is to be exercised both in prayer (beseeching God) and personal attention (beseeching humans). Both acts are the two parts of the overall commandment to attend to the needs of the sick (*biqur holim*).[21]

The treatment of those suffering from this disease is more for their sake than for the sake of the community in which they live. The community clearly has a responsibility for them, a responsibility involving both its physical and spiritual involvement. Furthermore, this concern is not limited to sufferers from the specific disease. In a parallel passage, the Talmud extends this procedure to those suffering from any other disease or misfortune as well.[22] Finally, once again emphasizing the general human problem involved in the AIDS problem, Jews are to be indiscriminate in terms of those who are the object of their medical attention, be they Jews or non-Jews.[23]

A serious problem does arise, however, when confronting the Talmud's rule that in the case of a "provocative sinner" (*mumar le-hakh'is*), one not only is not to help such a person but actually is not to save his or her life (*moridin ve-lo ma'alin*).[24] The question that must be honestly faced by all those who accept the authority of Jewish law, despite its obvious difficulty, is twofold: (1) whether the male homosexual or the drug user suffering from AIDS falls into this category, and (2) whether enforcement of the rule still applies under contemporary conditions.[25]

Regarding the first aspect, the provocative sinner is contrasted with the "sinner for appetite" (*mumar le-te'avon*). At first glance, it seems that because both active homosexuals and drug users apparently are motivated by "appetite," that their immediate gratification takes precedence over the observance of moral restraints. If this is the case, then the drastic action mandated by this Talmudic rule does not apply to them after all. However, the essential distinction between these two types of sinners is not seen to be the motivation behind their respective acts, that is, the former being motivated to rebel against the authority of God by violating what has been revealed in the Torah, and the latter being motivated by the desire for instant gratification. Rather, Maimonides interprets the difference between the two types of sinners to be whether the sin is habitual and willful or not.[26] If one sins habitually and willfully, then he or she is considered to be a *provocative* sinner. On the other hand, if one sins occasionally and with guilt, then he or she is considered to be a sinner *for appetite*. Actually, the term *appetite* is used here as an euphemism for weakness of will. The Talmudic way of describing such a person is that "he would not eat nonkosher food if kosher food were readily at hand."[27]

By this criterion, active homosexuals and drug users seem to fall into the category of provocative sinners. Their actions seem to be both habitual and willful. Furthermore, the recent attempt of some religious apologists for homosexuality to see active homosexuals as being under the influence of an unavoidable compulsion (*ones*) and thus not morally culpable is rationally flawed,[28] for it confuses the state of homosexual desire (or desire for drugs, if one is to follow this same logic) with homosexual activity. The Torah prohibits only homosexual activity, not homosexual desire, which can hardly be the subject of conscious choice.[29] Of course, because the presence of such desire makes avoidance of proscribed homosexual acts quite difficult, one could argue for the moral counsel that someone who is continually experiencing it seek professional help in order to sublimate it or, optimally, to experience heterosexual desire.[30] To assume that homosexual activity is as consciously involuntary as homosexual feeling and desire is to classify all homosexuals as being deprived of free choice. But that is hardly compassion, for it denies them their moral personality, an essential part of their full human function.[31] It erroneously assumes that only heterosexuals can separate sexual desire and sexual activity.

The designation of homosexuality as provocative sin has profound implications for understanding its essence from a Jewish point of view, as well as its current manifestation in connection with AIDS.

Because of the growing epidemic among heterosexuals (especially in Africa and Asia), there has been a concerted effort to deny any essential connection between AIDS and homosexuality. In terms of a specific connection, this argument is correct. AIDS is transmitted by heterosexual acts, just as it is transmitted by homosexual acts. But the argument misses the general, deeper point: AIDS is mostly transmitted by sexually promiscuous persons, whose very socially irresponsible promiscuity leaves them open to a whole series of infections, most seriously, but not exclusively, AIDS. The fact is that male homosexuals as a group are probably the most sexually promiscuous segment of our society. Hence, one can see AIDS as a problem primarily for the sexually promiscuous—both homosexual and heterosexual, but especially for homosexuals.

The question is why homosexuals are so promiscuous. Is their promiscuity essential to their homosexuality? There is good reason to believe so precisely because homosexuality cannot be socially structured into a procreative familial relationship, which Judaism has certainly seen as the foundation of society. The family is as much human society's connection to created nature as it is created nature's connection to human society.[32] In consequence, homosexuality is ultimately answerable only to the fulfillment of its immediate desire. It cannot essentially limit itself because it itself is not answerable to any greater order in which it participates. That is why, it seems to me, the Rabbis considered homosexuality to be an epitome of sin.[33] If humans are to rule over sin (Genesis 4:7), that rule must begin with the control of their own bodies, with what the Rabbis termed "conquering one's libido" (*ha-kovesh et yitsro*).[34] This is why, it seems to me, habitual and committed homosexuals are considered to be motivated by more than "appetite." It is not that they have succumbed to appetite; rather, they have constituted their very identity in it.

However, despite the fact that according to traditional criteria, active homosexuals are provocative sinners, even provocative sinners are capable of repentance, and repentance can thus be expected of them.[35] That still requires our respect; those deprived of free choice, on the other hand, can be the objects only of our pity. Our obligation, then, to care for AIDS patients, even if their disease is the result of grave sin, must not only tend to their bodies but respect their souls. Even the soul of the sinner is of infinitely greater importance than his or her sin.[36]

Despite the fact that many AIDS patients do fall into the category of the provocative sinner, there are times when the sanctions entailed by sin are not enforced.[37] In the Middle Ages, it was questioned why all provocative sinners are not included in the category of those whose lives are not to be saved. In fact, it was noted that the rule itself seems to be inconsistent, for it actually includes certain persons guilty of relatively minor sins and excludes other persons guilty of much more grave sins. One exegete explained this seeming inconsistency by noting that the criterion of inclusion is not due to the inherent nature per se of the proscribed acts being performed but, rather, to the likely consequences the Rabbis thought would result from issuing such a harsh warning.[38] Thus if the Rabbis thought that a relatively minor offense was being treated too lightly by the people, and that the threat of such a severe punishment would have a sobering effect on them, they enacted such a harsh sanction. This is seen as being justified by the power given to contemporary rabbinical authorities to exercise judgments more severe than those actually mandated by statute, if and when they deemed a situation in public morality an emergency.[39] So this category is subject to a high degree of judicial discretion.

Furthermore, it seems that by the time of the Middle Ages, the category of those whose lives are not to be saved was almost exclusively confined to persons whose deeds actually endangered the lives and property of the entire community, most notably, informers (*mosrim*). Along these lines, it seems that this type of reaction could conceivably apply to the AIDS patients who, despite their awareness of their highly contagious condition, still engage in sexual activity with unknowing partners. In the case of other AIDS patients, however, such sanctions, or even the threat of such sanctions, would be counterproductive. In modern times, this latter conclusion was powerfully formulated by the influential Israeli Talmudist and jurist R. Abraham Isaiah Karelitz (d. 1953), known as the Hazon Ish. He insisted that the purpose of all such rabbinic legislation is only to be constructive, a matter dependent on a judicial consideration of the times.[41]

The Question of Danger to Health Care Personnel

One of the moral problems that has arisen in connection with the AIDS crisis is the refusal of many health care personnel to treat AIDS patients at all. They argue that not only is AIDS highly contagious but the actual means of its contagion have by no means been ascertained. Without such definition, there is no real containment within predictable boundaries. Hence, the only sure way of not contracting the disease is to avoid any contact whatsoever with those who have AIDS. The question, then, is to what extent may the religiously based duty of self-preservation be invoked as prior to the religiously based duty to treat the sick, especially when one has unique skills for this through professional training.[42]

A truly adequate approach to this problem must begin with the question of what is the source of the obligation to treat the sick. This can be the only proper context for dealing with the more specific question of what is required of us in treating AIDS patients. In the classical Jewish sources there are two main theories concerning the source of the obligation to extend treatment to the sick: that of Maimonides (d. 1204), and that of Nahmanides (d. 1267).

In an early work, Maimonides argues that the obligation of the physician (*rofe*—which in our day can certainly be extended to all health care personnel) is derived from the fact that the scriptural law requiring that we return a lost article to its owner (Deuteronomy 22:2) is extended by the Talmud to include "returning his body to him," that is, saving his life.[43] In a later work, he reiterates the scriptural command, "You shall not stand idly by the blood of your neighbor" (Leviticus 19:16), which the Talmud connects with the previous interpretation of returning lost property (including a "lost" body) to its owner.[44] The latter verse is seen as being needed to teach the obligation to engage in such saving action even if it entails considerable effort and expense.

Even though Maimonides does not mention the actual duty of a physician in this later text, one can clearly extend the point made in it to include the physician. And, in regard to our problem of to what extent are health care personnel obligated to treat AIDS patients who do place them at some risk, the most important commentator on Maimonides, R. Joseph Karo (d. 1575), connects this text with an obscure rabbinic text that states that one is required to "expose himself to possible danger" (*safeq sakkanah*) when saving a human life.[45] Needless to say, the difference between "possible" danger and "definite" danger (*sakkanah vad'ai*) can be determined only on an *ad hoc* basis.

There are a number of problems with basing the duty to care for the sick on Maimonides' theory, and especially the duty to care for AIDS patients on it. First, the connection of the duty to extend oneself to someone in physical danger with the duty to expose oneself to possible danger is highly tenuous. Moreover, later commentators have great trouble altogether finding the rabbinic text that mandates exposure to possible danger. It is said to be from the Palestinian Talmud, but the great Talmudist R. Naftali Berlin (*Netsiv*, d. 1893) could find only a text there that deals with an individual's volunteering to risk his life for that of another.[46] Clearly, the permission and even the encouragement of a supererogatory act by a heroic individual cannot be the basis for a general norm requiring everyone in a similar situation to do so.[47]

Second, all of the Talmudic sources deal with situations where one *happens* to encounter other persons in dangerous situations. None of them deals with any obligation to choose and to remain in a health care profession and regularly treat all patients indiscriminately, for there such encounters are *regular* occurrences, not *chance happenings*. This is not to say that Maimonides himself, who was a distinguished physician, did not regard his profession of medicine to be a *vocatio;* from his biographical testimony we know that he did.[48] However, his theory of the obligation to extend medical care, indeed to choose to become a professional who regularly does so for better and for worse, does not seem to explain this obligation sufficiently.

To many students of Maimonides' writings, it has seemed quite odd that he did not quote or even paraphrase the well-known Talmud text that states, "It was taught in the School of R. Ishmael that from Scripture's words, 'he shall surely provide for his healing' [Exodus 21:19] is derived the permission for a physician to heal."[49] Perhaps Maimonides believed that the use of the term "permission" (*reshut*) indicated that such activity is only *optional;* therefore, the *obligation* to heal requires a stronger scriptural and Talmudic ground.[50] Nevertheless, Nahmanides (who was Maimonides' most cogent legal and theological critic) does quote this very text, and his exposition of it shows another theory, one that I believe is more adequate to the task at hand, both in terms of Jewish law and in terms of Jewish theology. The key difference between his theory and that of Maimonides is that he does not base the obligation to heal on an analogy between human life and human property, as does Maimonides.[51] Nahmanides writes:

> The explanation of this Talmud text is that the physician might say, "Why do I need this trouble; perhaps I might make a mistake [*et'eh*] and the result be that I have killed lives through error [*bi-shegagah*]?"; therefore, the Torah authorizes him [*natnah lo reshut*] to heal. . . . [T]here are

those who say that the physician is like a judge who is obligated to judge [*metsuveh la-doon*]. . . . And it makes sense . . .
also that they should not say, "God wounds and He heals"
since . . . human beings have become accustomed to medical
treatment [*be-refu'ot . . . she-nahagu*]. . . . Here "permission"
[*reshut*] means an obligation [*reshut de-mitsvah*] . . . which
God has designated for him to do.[52]

Here "permission" is not taken in its usual sense of that which
is optional but, rather, it is taken negatively, namely, that which
is not prohibited.[53] It is an authorization to perform a commandment, one that one might think is for God alone to do.

Nahmanides' analogy between a physician and a judge lies at
the heart of the theological point he is making here. In both professions, namely, those of healing and judging, the activity is
regarded as essentially divine and human only by participation.
Thus Scripture assures the judges that they should not be
deterred by the fact that their efforts have only partial results in
this world; indeed, it could not be otherwise because justice is
essentially transcendent.[54] "You shall not fear any man for judgment is God's" (Deuteronomy 1:17).[55]

God is also designated by Scripture as a physician. "Every
disease which I placed in Egypt I shall not place on you, for I the
Lord am your physician [*rof'ekha*]" (Exodus 15:26).[56] Just as, ideally, God should be the only judge, so, ideally, God should be the
only physician.[57] However, it is the less than ideal conditions of
human life on earth that require human judges and, for Nahmanides, especially require human physicians.[58] Nevertheless,
these human physicians must always appreciate their essentially subordinate role in the true created order.[59]

Nahmanides' theory of the obligation to heal makes it not just
an ordinary obligation but, rather, an act of *imitatio Dei*.[60] Indeed,
what for the Rabbis are the two main attributes of God, that of
judgment (*Elohim* qua *middat ha-din*) and that of compassion
(*YHWH* qua *middat rahamim*), can be seen as the basis for the
participatory status of judges and physicians: judges in the
attribute of judgment; physicians (and all other "healers") in the
attribute of compassion.

In terms of the obligation to treat AIDS patients, this is a crucial point, for AIDS is a disease, which at least for the time being,

allows its sufferers only to be treated, not cured. No one's life, now anyway, can be "saved." We can only *care for* these lives in the little time they have left. This requires greater effort; it also entails greater frustration because the ideology of modern medicine, like so much of the ideology of our technological civilization, is totally success oriented. We always want lasting results for our efforts, and here there are none. Yet Judaism obligates care, not just cure.[62] Here is where understanding our obligation as a divine commandment, one that is uniquely grounded in divine example, not just divine decree, alone makes sense of it, for it requires the infinite expenditure of compassion rather than the efficacy needed for finite results. That is why it cannot be an ordinary commandment, one simply based on divine decree.[63] This is important, too, for justifying treatment that only palliates (alleviating suffering as much as possible) rather than cures a disease, something that is clearly not the case at present with AIDS patients. In Maimonides' medical model, based as it is on the analogy of returning a lost piece of property, however, we are dealing with a case where a problem (a lost piece of property) is actually solved (it is returned to its owner). By contrast, Nahmanides' medical model explains only *care* of the sick, even when there can be no successful completion of a procedure.

The true results of our obedience to the commandments, the recompense for our exposure to toil and even danger in order to keep them, we are taught, lies in a realm beyond our experience and certainly beyond our grasp.[64] Hence, we can care for the AIDS patients because their imminent mortality does not catch us unaware. The commandments are addressed to us as equally mortal persons; we would not need them if we were anything else.[65] And the commandments save us from ultimate despair, which in the case of treating AIDS patients is such a strong and ever-present temptation. It saves us from despair because we are involved through the commandments in the very life of God himself, in which life, not death, is the final victor.[66]

Notes

1.   Re the debate on this subject, see M. A. Fumento, "AIDS: Are Heterosexuals at Risk?" *Commentary* 84 (1987): 21 ff.

2. Re hedonism and Judaism, see David Novak, *Halakhah in a Theological Dimension* (Chico, Calif., 1985), pp. 80–81.

3. See David Novak, *Jewish Social Ethics* (Oxford, 1992), pp. 135 ff.

4. The persistence of this question alone explains the enormous popularity of Harold Kushner's book, *When Bad Things Happen to Good People* (New York, 1981). However, Rabbi Kushner's conclusion, viz., that these things *happen* rather than being *caused* by God (see esp. pp. 113 ff.), is hardly consistent with the emphasis of traditional Jewish theology that everything other than our own free response to God is indeed "in the hands of God" (see *B. Berakhot* 33a and parallels re Deut. 10:12), and, as we shall soon see in this chapter, according to that theology, none of us can claim to be "good people."

5. The disturbing message of this verse (Exod. 20:5 and 34:7; Num. 14:18; Deut. 5:9) already troubled the prophets (see Jer. 31:28, Ezek. 18:2 ff.). The Talmud, in one comment, tries to qualify the message by stating that it applies only "when the children hang onto [i.e., willfully repeat] the deeds of their parents" (*B. Berakhot* 7a, *B. Sanhedrin* 27b). Nevertheless, the fact that children do suffer because of their parents' misdeeds is too apparent ever to be fully explained away. See, e.g., *Y. Megillah* 4.12/75d and esp. R. Samuel David Luzzatto (Shadal), *Commentary on the Torah*, Exod. 20:5; also Novak, *Halakhah in a Theological Dimension*, pp. 11 ff.

6. See Gen. 8:21; also Solomon Schechter, *Some Aspects of Rabbinic Theology* (New York, 1936), pp. 242 ff., and Will Herberg, *Judaism and Modern Man* (New York, 1951), pp. 74 ff.

7. See David Novak, *Law and Theology in Judaism*, 2 vols. (New York, 1974–76), 1:1 ff., 2:xiii ff.

8. See *B. Yebamot* 76a; Maimonides, *Hilkhot Isuray Bi'ah* 21:8; also David Novak, *The Image of the Non-Jew in Judaism: An Historical and Constructive Study of the Noahide Laws* (New York, 1983), pp. 213–215.

9. *B. Sanhedrin* 57b re Lev. 18:6. For a fuller discussion of the prohibition of homosexuality, see Novak, *Jewish Social Ethics*, pp. 89 ff.

10. *B. Sanhedrin* 58a.

11. See David Novak, *Jewish-Christian Dialogue: A Jewish Justification* (New York, 1989), introduction.

12. *B. Baba Kama* 91b.

13. *B. Avodah Zarah* 18a. See *B. Berakhot* 32b re Deut. 4:9, 15.

14. See *B. Sanhedrin* 46b.

15. *B. Baba Batra* 17a. See *B. Yevamot* 103b and parallels with Maharsha, *Hiddushay Aggadot* ad loc.; *Wisdom of Solomon* 2:24; Nahmanides, *Torat Ha'Adam*, Sha'ar Ha-Gemul, introduction, in *Kitvay Ramban*, 2 vols., ed. C. B. Chavel (Jerusalem, 1963), 2:12.

16. *B. Berakhot* 5a–b.

17. *The Authorised Daily Prayer Book*, ed. S. Singer (London, 1962), p. 353. See *M. Sanhedrin* 6:2; *B. Shabbat* 32b; Nahmanides, *Torat Ha'Adam*, Inyan Viduy, *Kitvay Ramban*, 2:47; *Shulhan Arukh*, Yoreh De'ah 338:2.

18. See, e.g., *T. Nega'im* 6.7; *Arakhin* 15b re Lev. 14:2.

19.   See *Arakhin* 16b re Lev. 13:46. However, it is important to note that the Rabbis regarded *tsara'at*'s contagion to be moral rather than physical. See, e.g., *M. Nega'im* 3.2; Malmonides, *Hilkhot Tum'at Tsara'at* 9:8.

20.   *B. Mo'ed Qatan* 5a. Cf. Maimonides, *Hilkhot Tum'at Tsara'at* 10:8.

21.   See *B. Nedarim* 39b–40a.

22.   *B. Sotah* 32b; *Shulhan Arukh*, Yoreh De'ah 335:8.

23.   See *B. Gittin* 61a.

24.   *B. Avodah Zarah* 26b.

25.   Theoretically, a rabbinic law (such as this one) can be repealed (see *M. Eduyot* 1:5); however, in actual practice, reexamination of the conditions required for the application of the law was the usual procedure for effecting change. See, e.g., *M. Kiddushin* 4:14; *B. Kiddushin* 82a; Karo, *Shulhan Arukh*, Even Ha'Ezer 24:1 and Sirkes, *Bach* on *Tur*, Even Ha'Ezer 24; also Karo, *Kesef Mishneh* on Maimonides, *Hilkhot Tefillah* 11:1.

26.   *Hilkhot Rotseah* 4:10 and *Hilkhot Teshuvah* 3:9 (see Karo, *Kesef Mishneh* ad loc.); also *Hilkhot Yesoday Ha-Torah* 5:10.

27.   *Hullin* 4a and parallels. For eating as a euphemism for sexual activity, see *Semahot* 7:8 and *B. Kiddushin* 21b–22a.

28.   See H. J. Matt, "An Approach to Homosexuality," *Judaism* 27 (1978): 16.

29.   See Norman Lamm, "Judaism and the Modern Attitude to Homosexuality," *Encyclopaedia Judaica Yearbook: 1974*, pp. 194 ff. For further background, see Samuel H. Dresner, "Homosexuality and the Order of Creation," *Judaism* 40 (1991): 309–321.

30.   See David Novak, "On Homosexuality," *Sh'ma*, 11/201 (Nov. 14, 1980), pp. 3–5.

31.   See Maimonides, *Hilkhot Teshuvah* 4:1 ff.

32.   See Novak, *Jewish Social Ethics*, p. 87.

33.   See ibid., p. 90. For the authoritative view that all nonmarital sex is sinful, see *Sifre*, Devarim, no. 260 re Deut. 23:18; Maimonides, *Hilkhot Ishut* 1:4 and R. Vidal of Tolosa, *Maggid Mishneh* ad loc.

34.   See *M. Avot* 4:1 re Prov. 16:32; *B. Avodah Zarah* 19a re Ps. 112:1; *B. Sanhedrin* 19b–20a.

35.   See Maimonides, *Hilkhot Teshuvah* 7:1 ff.

36.   For the refusal to equate the sinner with his or her sin, see *B. Berakhot* 10a re Ps. 104:35.

37.   See *B. Betsah* 28b. For the whole problem of the administration of punishment in Jewish law, see M. Elon, *Ha-Mishpat Ha'Ivri*, 2 vols., 2nd ed. (Jerusalem, 1978), 1:421 ff.

38.   R. Joseph ibn Habib, *Nimuqey Yosef* on *B. Avodah Zarah* 26b, ed. Blau, 203, in the name of *Tosfot Ha-R'osh*. Also see *Tosfot Rabbenu Samson of Sens* ad loc., ed. Blau, 82.

39.   See *B. Sanhedrin* 46a; also Maimonides, *Hilkhot Sanhedrin* 24:10.

40.   See *Responsa Ha-R'osh*, ed. Venice (1552), 17:1.

41. *Hazon Ish,* Yoreh De'ah (B'nai B'rak, 1958), sec. 2, 7d. Cf. *B. Gittin* 33a, Tos., s.v. *v'afqa'inhu.*

42. See *Sifra,* Behar re Lev. 25:36, ed. Weiss, 199c; *B. Baba Metsia* 62a.

43. *Commentary on the Mishnah,* Nedarim 4:4.

44. *Hilkhot Rotseah* 1:14 elaborating on *B. Sanhedrin* 73a.

45. See Karo, *Kesef Mishneh* on Maimonides, *Hilkhot Rotseah;* also Karo, *Bet Yosef* on *Tur,* Hoshen Mishpat 426 re Lev. 19:16 and *M. Sanhedrin* 4.5. Along similar lines, see *B. Baba Metsia* 30b re Exod. 18:20; R. Solomon Luria, *Yam Shel Shlomoh, Baba Kama* 6:26 re *B. Baba Kama* 60b. Cf., however, R. David ibn Abi Zimra, *Responsa Ha-Radbaz,* 3, no. 627; R. Joshua Falk, *Me'irat Aynayim* on *Shulhan Arukh,* Hoshen Mishpat 426.

46. *Ha'Ameq Sh'elah* on *She'iltot de-Rav Hai Gaon,* Shelah, end re *Y. Terumot* 8:4/46b. Viktor Aptowitzer argued in his "Unechte Jeruschalmizitate," *Monatsschrift für Geschichte und Wissenschaft des Judenthums* 55 (1911): 419 ff., and on this point he has been followed by other modern critical Talmudists, that when a medieval source quotes the Yerushalmi and we do not have this source in our Yerushalmi text, then the citation may very well be from a now-lost rabbinic collection (*Qovetz Yerushalmi* or *Sefer Yerushalmi*). See also R. Zvi Hirsch Chajes' note on *B. Megillah* 12b, and *Imray Binah,* sec. 2 in *Kol Sifray Maharats Chajes,* 2 vols. (B'nai B'rak, 1958), 2:891 ff.

47. See J. Halberstam, "Supererogation in Jewish *Halakhah* and Islamic *Shari'a,*" in *Studies in Islamic and Jewish Traditions,* ed. W. M. Brinner and S. D. Ricks (Atlanta, 1986), pp. 85 ff.

48. See my late revered teacher Abraham Joshua Heschel, *Maimonides: A Biography,* trans. J. Neugroschel (New York, 1982), pp. 213 ff.

49. *B. Baba Kama* 85a.

50. See, e.g., *B. Berakhot* 27b; Maimonides, *Hilkhot Tefillah* 1:6. For the attempt to see *reshut* as designating a low level of obligation rather than a pure option, see *M. Betsah* 5:2 and *B. Betsah* 36b; *B. Berakhot* 26a, Tos., s.v. *ta'ah;* ibid., 27b, Tos., s.v. *halakhah.* Regardless of which interpretation one accepts, however, the term *reshut* is not strong enough to ground the sense of *vocatio* needed for the practice of medicine as a profession.

51. For the pitfalls of using economic analogies when dealing with the protection of human persons, see R. Stith, "Toward Freedom from Value," *Jurist* 38 (1978): 48 ff.

52. *Torat Ha'Adam,* Inyan Ha-Sakanah, *Kitvey Ramban* 2:41–43. See also David Novak, *The Theology of Nahmanides: Systematically Presented* (Atlanta, 1992).

53. For *reshut* in this stronger sense, see esp. R. Joshua Falk, *Perishah* on *Tur,* Yoreh De'ah 336, n. 4.

54. See *M. Avot* 2:16; Novak, *Jewish Social Ethics,* pp. 163 ff.

55. See *B. Sanhedrin* 6b.

56. For God's greater healing power than man's, see *Mekhilta,* Be-Shelah, ed. Horovitz-Rabin, 156.

57. For uneasiness with human authority in relation to divine authority, see Jud. 8:22–23, I Sam. 8:5 ff.

58. See, e.g., Nahmanides, *Commentary on the Torah*, Lev. 26:11.

59. For a powerful theological statement against the prevailing medical absolutism of this secular age, see my late friend Paul Ramsey, *The Patient as Person* (New Haven, 1970), pp. 115, 156–157.

60. See *B. Shabbat* 133b re Exod. 15:2; *Beresheet Rabbah* 8, end.

61. See A. Marmorstein, *The Old Rabbinic Doctrine of God*, 2 vols. (New York, 1968), 1:43 ff.

62. See *B. Yoma* 85a; *B. Yevamot* 80a–b, and Rashi, s.v. *mipnay sakkanah*; *B. Shabbat* 151b; *B. Nedarim* 39b (the retort of R. Aha bar Hanina); Sirkes, *Bach* on *Tur*, Hoshen Mishpat 426 re the limitations of the Maimonidean model for medical treatment.

63. See *B. Sotah* 14a re Gen. 18:1; *B. Baba Kama* 99b–100a re Exod. 18:20.

64. *B. Kiddushin* 39b. See *B. Berakhot* 34b re Isa. 64:3.

65. See *B. Kiddushin* 54a; *Shir Ha-Shirim Rabbah* 8:13 re Num. 19:14.

66. See *B. Pesahim* 68b.

An Analysis of Some Social Issues Related to HIV Disease from the Perspective of Jewish Law and Values (1990)

Benjamin Freedman

Jewish law (*halakha*) and its associated literature comprise one of the oldest and most developed systems for the analysis of bioethical issues. For a number of reasons, however, this resource has rarely been utilized by secular philosophers and ethicists (in sharp contrast to the Roman Catholic tradition, although the latter is itself intrinsically as parochial and logically reliant upon specific religious commitments as is Judaism).

Jewish legal literature has been inaccessible because of the language in which it is written and the lack of an authoritative, canonical formulation, among other technical barriers to scholarly use. Equally daunting, perhaps, has been the specific methodology used in reasoning through a problem to its ethical conclusion. The rabbinic vocabulary of ethical concepts presumes familiarity with deontic schemata (rules, intercorrelated collections of rules, and value statements) derived from biblical injunctions and descriptions (together with their associated traditional exegesis) as well as analogical reasoning from concrete puzzle cases described in the Mishna and the Talmuds.

The familiar difficulties in analogical reasoning—closeness of the analogy, conflicting analogies, etc.—are compounded in a number of ways when considering Jewish approaches to the ethical issues posed by human immunodeficiency virus (HIV) disease and its late, fatal stage, acquired immunodeficiency syndrome (AIDS). First, although Jewish law has dealt with ethical issues arising during infectious disease epidemics (notably including obligations to protect community health and to arrange care for disease victims),[1] the conclusions then reached cannot be mechanically applied to the current situation. Earlier plagues, for example, usually involved less lethal pathogens; at the same time, the risk of contagion was far higher, was unavoidable given then-current knowledge and techniques, and involved a much higher degree of uncertainty than at present. Accounts of conduct during earlier plagues are in some respects not therefore normatively relevant to AIDS. Jewish approaches to AIDS are further complicated because the concrete puzzle cases that serve as the common focus of discussion in Jewish legal reasoning have an antique character (as a result of their Talmudic, or even biblical, origin). This raises a problem of distance between them and our familiar ethical questions and associated categories.

An example will help to demonstrate the difficulty involved in using Jewish legal reasoning to consider AIDS. At some point, providers of health care to HIV-infected patients may claim a right to a risk increment in their pay (a position with historical precedent).[2] Rabbinic Judaism's perspective is more one of duty and obligation than of rights. From its point of view, we shall need to ask whether an individual is permitted, in the interest of remuneration, to undergo a small increment in physical harm or risk. The relevant concrete puzzle case is an anecdote told of Rav Chisda.[3] When Rav Chisda would walk among thorns he would protect his garment by lifting it, for his skin would heal but his garment could not repair itself. Some 1,600 years later, the case was cited by Rabbi Zvi Beer as authority for the proposition that self-mutilation is permissible when undertaken to avoid monetary loss.[4]

These theoretical difficulties are illustrated in the following discussions of (1) the relationship between ethics, sin, and illness, raising issues of biblical ethics; (2) confidentiality and privacy issues and the problems associated with the unfamiliarity of the rabbinic ordering of values; and (3) the duty to care for the sick and dying, expressed in Talmudic literature through concrete anecdotes requiring abstract extrapolation.

In spite of these difficulties, there appear to be directions of thought within the Jewish tradition that can help to determine a proper perspective upon the issue at hand, and a perspective that is distinctively Jewish. First, Judaism has, throughout history, emphasized the importance of maintaining the highest level of community safety and individual health. The sources for this date back to the biblical era and are expressed in the command *v'nishmartem m'od l'nafshoteichem*, to take good heed of your health.[5] Further indications of this concern for safety and health are found in such *mitzvot* (religious commandments) as the requirement that a homeowner construct a parapet for his or her roof[6] and the jurisdiction granted to traditional Jewish courts (*batei din*) to establish and enforce edicts protecting community health.[1] The basic principle has been that concerns for safety take precedence over other religious obligations (*chamura sakanata me'issura*).

Second, Judaism has always seen duties toward the ill as community responsibilities rather than private concerns. For example, Jews emphasize the continuing presence of the sick within the community by praying for the ill *betokh sh'ar cholei Yisrael*, in the midst of the other ill *within* Israel.[7]

Sin and Illness

In some Christian fundamentalist circles, discussion of the ethical and policy issues arising from HIV disease has been commonly predicated upon the presumptive sinfulness of those acquiring the infection. Within rabbinic Judaism, both male homosexual activity and illegal intravenous drug use—the major routes of HIV exposure in North America—are similarly sinful activities, and some Jewish discussions have been dominated by the issues of sin and illness, as in the list of issues posed by one well-known writer:

> Should a Jewish drug addict who develops AIDS as a result of sinful activity be treated any differently than any other patient? Should the Jewish homosexual who develops AIDS . . . be treated? Does Judaism teach compassion for all who suffer illness irrespective of whether or not the illness is the result of practices which Judaism abhors and prohibits? . . . Should the Jewish community expend resources for AIDS research and treatment, since most such patients are sinners? Should not the resources better be allocated to the health of law-abiding citizens? Can patients with AIDS be counted in a quorum of ten men?[8]

Even if HIV transmission involved sinful activity, the actor's status as a sinner does not follow. A sinful act perpetrated under conditions of duress—including overpowering psychological compulsion—remains sinful, but its perpetrator falls within the excused rabbinic category of *ones*.[9] In the absence of excusable psychological compulsion, reasoning from the status of the act to that of the actor is impossible because of the possibility that the actor repented. In the case of suicide, these two possibilities in combination have gained the force of a rebuttable legal presumption that the actor was not culpable.

Analysis at a much more basic level reveals a radical dichotomy in the Judaic attitude toward illness, one that can be traced to biblical roots. Even though illness is closely associated with sin, Judaism nonetheless recognizes moral duties to the ill. Within the Bible, illness is commonly described as punishment for sin, with no corresponding diminishment of obligations toward the ill. Moses's sister, Miriam, is struck with leprosy as punishment for having spoken ill of him; he prays for her recovery.[10] The congregation of Israel is consumed by a plague for murmuring rebellion against Moses and Aaron, and Aaron runs, at Moses's instruction, to contain the plague.[11]

Within Judaism, duties toward the ill are, paradoxically, not affected by the reason behind the illness, precisely because the connection between sin and illness is so strong. The traditional belief, rooted in the Bible,[12] was that illness is both caused and sustained by sin: "R. Alexandrai said that R. Chiya bar Aba said,

'The sick one does not stand apart from his sickness until all his sins are forgiven him.'"[13] Inasmuch as there exists this general presumption that illness is caused by sin, were there no duty to care for the *sinful* ill, the duty to care for the ill would never in fact obtain!

The normative barrier between the cause of illness and duties toward the ill is indeed so strong that the fact may not even be mentioned to the sufferer:

> Included in the sin of verbal oppression is shaming one's neighbor by words in private; much more so, shaming him thus in public or doing something to him which causes him to be ashamed in public. As stated in *Perek Hazahav*,[14] "if he is beset by sickness, one should not say to him as was said to Job by his friends,[15] "Remember, which clean man is destroyed?"[16]

Confidentiality and Rabbinic Valuation

Perhaps the single most discussed ethical issue associated with HIV disease is confidentiality and the right to privacy. Secular bioethical concern and analyses have centered around professional—specifically, medical—confidentiality, which is distinct from the requirements of confidentiality in ordinary life in at least two ways. Professional confidentiality is commonly considered to impose a more stringent ethical obligation than does ordinary confidentiality (for example, the requirements of professional confidentiality may override the requirement to cooperate with the judicial system). Furthermore, knowledge gained through professional interactions is presumed to be confidential unless otherwise specified, whereas just the opposite presumption—that confidentiality is not required unless specifically requested—obtains in ordinary interactions.[17]

Neither characteristic of confidentiality holds within rabbinic Judaism. A specific professional duty of confidentiality is unrecognized, indeed, disallowed. The following excerpt, from a responsum by R. Joseph Colon, answers the claim that a pledge of professional confidentiality may override the obligation to proclaim the discovery of lost property:

> I have seen that if one takes an oath to disregard the laws of his community, such an oath is a nullity. If the oath-taker

had received proper warning [of this illegality], he is liable to corporal punishment under biblical law. The man is not excused from the community ordinance, even though his oath preceded the promulgation of the ordinance. He has taken an oath to nullify a divine commandment, i.e., to depart from the commanded statutes. On this score every Jew is deemed to be under oath from the time of the Revelation on Mount Sinai.[18]

At the same time, Jewish rules respecting ordinary confidentiality—addressed under the rubrics of "talebearing" (*lashon hara* and *r'khilut*)—are presumed to apply unless a specific exemption from the duty has been granted by the one supplying the information.[19] The deep rigor and detailed regulations governing confidentiality in ordinary Jewish social interchange correspond to the secular professional cognate. And the presumption is that these strictures obtain unless an explicit exemption has been granted. Roughly speaking, therefore, it might be argued that these two Jewish deviations from the common secular understanding of confidentiality cancel each other out. Although professional morality is not granted privileged and stringent status, within Judaism ordinary confidentiality itself approaches the stringency associated with professional confidentiality.

The dilemmas associated in secular ethics with the protection of professional confidentiality are therefore reproduced within Judaism in the context of community interaction. Perhaps the most familiar such dilemma concerns the justification of a violation of confidentiality necessary to preserve the interests of a third party. Secular bioethics asks whether a doctor has a duty or even a privilege to warn an uninfected spouse of his or her partner's HIV infection. Most professional associations have asserted that confidentiality may indeed be violated in these circumstances.[20]

A normatively identical problem arises within Jewish thought for any individual, professional or layperson, who learns of a disqualification of marriage in a prospective bridegroom. Must the fiancee be informed of such a fact about her affianced? Or is the disclosure of such a fact barred by the stringent Jewish prohibitions against talebearing? An extended discussion of such a case is found in the work of Rabbi Israel Meir Hacohen (epony-mously known as the Chafetz Chaim after the title of one of his many volumes on the laws of talebearing). The author states that disclosure is permitted—is in fact mandatory—provided that several requirements have been satisfied. As applied to the case of an HIV-infected spouse, these requirements might be under-stood as follows:

1. *The information is known to be accurate.* For example, one must have taken more than ordinary care to ensure confirmatory HIV testing of the spouse and to exclude the possibility of labo-ratory error and erroneous interpretation of an ambiguous result.

2. *There is no other alternative that will prevent the harm.* For example, the infected spouse has specifically refused to disclose this fact to his wife and has either refused to confine their sexual intercourse to safe practices or has shown himself to be unreli-able in that regard.

3. *The harm may be prevented by telling.* If, in the scenario of the prospective bridegroom, one knows that the marriage will not be broken off despite the disclosure (e.g., because the informer will not be believed), the warrant for disclosure is lacking.[21] Sim-ilarly, if one were certain that the spouse would not believe or would refuse to act upon the information provided, a violation of confidentiality would be otiose and would accordingly be prohibited.

4. *The information is not represented in overly dramatic or exagger-ated form.* Given the fear that the informer may be disregarded, there exists a temptation to convey the information in an omi-nous manner, to ensure that the spouse will heed the warning. But the truth of the warning is a function of its form and manner as well as its content, and the obligation to warn does not carry with it the freedom to stretch the truth.

5. *The harms of disclosure are proportionate to those of nondisclo-sure.* A further requirement discussed by the Chafetz Chaim is equivocally stated and conceptually very complicated. In one quasi-utilitarian version, he states that the harm caused by vio-lating the confidence must be less than would have been caused by failing to violate the confidence. In another version of this cri-

terion, he writes that the harm that will be caused by violating the confidence must be no greater than what would be legally imposed when information about the misfeasance receives judicial notice.

This criterion has been applied in classical Jewish reasoning to the situation of informing a prospective business partner about the nature or liabilities of his counterpart. In this context, it requires that a degree of balance be established between the harms of disclosure and nondisclosure and that judicial notice and penalty serve as a measure of this balance. A reasonable balancing of the harms of disclosure against those of nondisclosure may seem to be in order in personal relations as well, but the problems of measuring and predicting harm are great, and perhaps insuperable, in the absence of an established burden of proof. This difficulty, it should be noted, has been mentioned in other discussions of confidentiality, for example, when LeRoy Walters[22] discussed the balancing of harms as a basis for overriding the prima facie requirements of professional confidentiality.

Duties of Caring for the Sick and the Dying

The third methodological problem noted above was the difficulty in extrapolating abstract principles of duty and right action from the concrete cases and discussions found in Talmudic sources. This complication may be illustrated by reference to numerous homiletic and normative statements regarding duties to visit and care for the sick (generally noted within the rubric of *bikkur cholim*) and the dying. In the following Talmudic discussions of the duty to care for the ill,[23] we may discern and extrapolate a distinctive approach to illness that is all the more striking because it arises from a tradition and a time in which caring for the ill amounted primarily to comfort and fellowship rather than the provision of therapeutic intervention.

The Priority of Comforting and Visiting the Sick

We learned in a *b'raita:* "Visiting the sick has no measure." What is meant by "has no measure"? Rav Yosef thought to say that there is no measure to its reward. Abaye said to him, "And for all [other] *mitzvot* is there then a measure for reward? Insofar as we had learned in a *mishna*, 'Be as painstaking with a light *mitzva* as with a weighty one, for you know not the reward of *mitzvot*.'" But Ataye stated instead, "Even a great one visits a little one." Rava said, "Even a hundred times a day." . . . As Rav Chelbo became ill there was none who came to visit. He said to them, "Was this not as the story of one student amongst the students of Rabbi Akiva who became ill? The wise men did not enter, but Rabbi Akiva entered to visit him, and because he did so they entered and served before him and he lived, and said to him, 'Rabbi, you have sustained my life.'" Rabbi Akiva went out and taught, "Anyone who does not visit the sick is like one who spills blood."[24]

The Ill Person Retains Inalienable Dignity

It is otherwise for a sick person, for the Divine Presence (variant manuscripts: the Holy One, Blessed Be He) is with him, in accord with what was said by Rav Anan in the name of Rav:

> From whence do we learn that the Divine Presence cares for the welfare of the sick person? From the verse, "G-d shall [preserve us/care for us/nourish us; *yis'adenu*] upon the sick bed."[25] We have learned a *b'raita* in accord with this as well: "One who enters to visit the sick should not sit upon the bed nor upon a chair [variant texts add: and not upon a stool or a high place], but wraps himself [in his tallit] and sits before [and beneath] him, because the Divine Presence is above the head of the sick one, as it is written, 'G-d shall preserve us upon the sick bed.'"[26]

Sensitivity in Providing Care and Arranging Visitation

> Rav Sheisha, son of Rav Idi, said: "A person should not visit in the first three hours of the day, nor in the last three hours of the day, in order that he not neglect to ask mercy for him. For in the first three hours he [the sick person] is at ease [and does not seem to be in need of prayer], and in the last three hours he is overwhelmed by weakness [and appears to be hopeless]."[24]

This last rule shows a fine sensitivity to the interactive process between patient and caregiver. Another illustration is found in a rule restricting visits, though not care, to those suffering gastrointestinal complaints (for fear of embarrassing the sufferer) and eye ailments or headache (for fear of exacerbating their pain).[27]

These tales and discussions have served as the basis for extrapolated principles. The specific restriction on visiting those suffering gastric complaints is generalized by Maimonides[28] as a prohibition against a visitor's presence when caregivers are tending to the patient's physical needs. The *Shulchan Arukh*, an authoritative compendium of Jewish law, states in the most general fashion[29] that one may not visit the ill if the visit will be a burden or cause discomfort, but that, even so, one should attend to the person to see if there is some fashion in which one may be useful.

The difficulties of extrapolating from the concrete antique situations to abstract contemporary principles are obvious, but the necessity is inescapable, given the nature of Talmudic material. I would conclude by suggesting some reflections on appropriate care for those dying of AIDS, within or outside a hospice, drawn from remarks by Ben Azzai:

> If [at death] one fixes his gaze at men, it is good; if at the wall, it is bad; if one's face is bright, good; if one's face is overcast, bad; if with a clear mind, good; if deranged, bad; if while speaking, good; if in silence, bad; if while Torah is spoken, good; while business, bad; if while carrying out a *mitzva*, good; while engaged in an idle matter, bad; if in the midst of joy, good; in sadness, bad; if while laughing, good; while weeping, bad.[30]

Acknowledgments and Notes

My work on these questions was spurred by participation in the Ad Hoc Task Force on AIDS established by Allied Jewish Community Services of Montreal. I am grateful to the other committee members and especially to the chair, Dr. Harold Frank, for comments. Rabbi Reuben Poupko provided invaluable assistance. I am wholly responsible for any errors of fact or judgment.

All references to Hebrew materials represent the author's own translation.

This work was supported in part by Grant #6605-2897 from the National Health Research and Development Program, Ministry of Health, Government of Canada.

The author's work in Jewish medical ethics is greatly facilitated by the contribution of the Drazin family of Montreal, in the form of the Drazin Collection of Jewish Medical Ethics, reposed at the medical library of the Sir Mortimer B.

Davis–Jewish General Hospital of Montreal. I am deeply grateful to the family for providing this facility.

The editor records with sorrow the untimely death of Professor Benjamin Freedman (1951–1997). May his memory be blessed.

1. I. Jakobovits, *Jewish Medical Ethics* (New York: Bloch, 1959), especially chaps. 1, 3, 4, and 11.

2. D. M. Fox, "The Politics of Physicians' Responsibility in Epidemics: A Note on History," *Hastings Center Report* 8, suppl. (April–May 1988): 5–9.

3. Babylonian Talmud, Tractate *Bava Kamma* 91b.

4. A. Levine, *Free Enterprise and Jewish Law* (New York: Ktav, 1980).

5. Deuteronomy 4:15.

6. Deuteronomy 22:8. Compare Maimonides, *Mishne Tora, Hilkhot Rotzeach*, beginning at chapter 11:4.

7. "Our rabbis learned: One who enters to visit the sick says: 'Shabbat precludes beseechings [*shabbat hi miliz'ok*] and healing will come soon.' Rabbi Yose says: 'The Omnipresent shall have mercy upon you in the midst of the sick of Israel.' Whose approach is followed by Rabbi Chanina in his saying, 'One who has a sick one in his home must meld him within the midst of the sick of Israel.' Like whom?—like Rabbi Yose." Talmud Bavli, *Shabbat* 12a

8. F. Rosner, "AIDS: A Jewish View," *Journal of Halakha and Contemporary Society*, 13 (Spring 1987/Pesach 5741): 21–41. (In this volume, above, p. 96).

9. For a discussion of the complexities in this suggestion, as well as the analogy to halakhic developments with respect to suicide, see N. Lamm, "Judaism and the Modern Attitude to Homosexuality," in *Contemporary Jewish Ethics*, ed. M. M. Kellner (New York: Sanhedrin Press, 1978), pp. 375–399.

10. Numbers 12:13.

11. Numbers 17:6–15.

12. Compare Exodus 15:26.

13. Talmud Bavli, *N'darim* 41a.

14. Talmud Bavli, *Bava Metzia* 58b.

15. Job 4:7.

16. R. Moshe Chayim Luzzatto, *Msillat Ysharim*, trans. S. Silverstein, 2nd ed. (New York: Feldheim Publishers, 1966), "The Particulars of Cleanliness."

17. B. Freedman, "A Meta-Ethics for Professional Morality," *Ethics* 89, no. 1 (1978): 1–19.

18. Responsum of R. Joseph Colon (*Maharik*), no. 110, in *Jewish Law and Jewish Life: Selected Rabbinical Responsa*, ed. J. Bazak, trans. S. M. Passamaneck, Book 1: *Lawyers, Judges and Legal Ethics* (New York: Union of American Hebrew Congregations, 1977).

19. The Talmudic derivation of the rule regarding the presumption of confidentiality is somewhat fanciful: "Rav Musia, grandson of R. Musia, said in the name of R. Musia the greater: 'From whence do we learn that one who says something to his friend, [the latter] is prohibited to repeat it unless he tells

him to go and say it—as it says, "And G-d spoke to him from the tent of meeting to say [lemor]."""—*T.B. Yoma 4b*; Steinsaltz in his adjoining commentary indicates that the rule is codified in law in *Smag* and in *Magen Avraham*.

20.   The position of the Canadian Medical Association is typical. "The CMA advises physicians that disclosure to a spouse or current sexual partner may not be unethical and, indeed, may be indicated when physicians are confronted with an HIV-infected patient who is unwilling to inform the person at risk. Such disclosure may be justified when all of the following conditions are met: the partner is at risk of infection with HIV and has no other reasonable means of knowing of the risk; the patient has refused to inform his or her sexual partner; the patient has refused an offer of assistance by the physician to do so on the patient's behalf; and the physician has informed the patient of his or her intention to disclose the information to the partner" ("CMA Position: Acquired Immunodeficiency Syndrome," *Canadian Medical Association Journal* 140 [1989]: 64a).

21.   This provision is represented in the text by the requirement that the informer's motive be solely that of preventing the harm. The necessary formal test for validating that this is the informer's motivation is whether disclosure may serve to prevent the harm. The connection in Judaism between intention and potential consequences differs in important respects from the Catholic approach, in ways too complicated to pursue here.

22.   L. Walters, "Ethical Aspects of Medical Confidentiality," in *Contemporary Issues in Bioethics*, ed. T. L. Beauchamp and L. Walters (Encino, Calif.: Dickenson, 1978), pp. 169–175.

23.   See *Shulchan Arukh, Yoreh De'ah*, chap. 335; Talmud Bavli, *Shabbat* 12a.

24.   *Talmud Bavli, N'darim* 39b.

25.   Psalms 41:4.

26.   Psalms 41:4. Note there Tosfot, beginning "Shall not sit": "Apparently only when the sick person is laying in a low place, that he not sit higher than the head of the sick one."

27.   *Talmud Bavli, N'darim* 41a.

28.   *Mishne Torah, Hilchot Aivel* 14:5.

29.   *Yore De'ah* 335:8.

30.   *Avot deRabbi Nathan*, chap. 25.

Compulsory Testing and Treatment for AIDS (1989)

ﭏﭏ

Shlomo Deichowsky

AIDS—to this day, unfortunately, still an incurable disease—raises a number of halakhic issues, in addition to a wide range of medical and social problems. An essential issue relevant to AIDS is the identification of high-risk groups and the enforcement upon members of these groups of a test making it possible to ascertain whether they are carriers of the virus causing the disease. The test, which is performed on a simple blood specimen, is important for the tested person himself (even though there is as yet no cure for AIDS), and is even more important for everyone in contact with him.

There are two halakhic issues involved here:

1. May a patient be treated against his will?
2. May a person be forced to undergo medical treatment or testing whose aim is to prevent harm to others?

Compulsory Treatment

As is well known, Nachmanides (Ramban) opined that men of piety ought not to seek medical treatment. In his Biblical commentary he says:

> During the era of the prophets, the pious, if they happened to sin and fell ill, sought the counsel only of the prophets,

not of physicians. [This was] in contrast to the behavior of
Asa, of whom it is said: "Even in his illness he did not seek
the Lord, but the help of physicians" (II Chron. 16:12). . . .
When the Rabbis said that the verse "he shall surely heal"
(Ex. 21:19) indicates that physicians are permitted to heal,[1]
they did not imply thereby that patients are permitted to
seek human treatment. Rather, they meant to say that if a
patient *does* seek such treatment, as is common behavior,
rather than content himself with belonging to the
community of those of unrestricted piety [who rely on a
heavenly cure], then the physician should not refrain from
treating him. The physician may not refuse treatment either
with the argument that the patient may die during the treatment—for we assume that the physician is well trained—or
on the grounds that God alone heals all flesh.[2] . . . This is
why a person who injures another "by stone or fist" (Ex.
21:18) is obligated to pay for the cure: indeed, the laws of
the Torah do not rely on miracles. . . . Still, if a man's conduct pleases God, he has no need whatsoever for medical
treatment.[3]

Rashba and the *Tur* seem to express a contrary opinion: "'he
shall surely heal'—this clearly implies that the physician is permitted to heal. . . . This is an obligation [for the physician], and it
is a part of one's duty to save life (*piqquah nefesh*)."[4]

The *Bayit Hadash* adds ad loc.:

Does not the verse about Asa, stating "Even in his illness he
did not seek the Lord, but the help of physicians" (II Chron.
16:12), imply that it is prohibited to seek medical treatment
for a blow inflicted by Heaven? No; rather, it is because he
[Asa] sought help *only* from physicians, and *none* from God,
that he was punished. However, if one puts his trust in God
to heal him by means of the physician, then he is allowed to
seek medical advice, even in order to provide a cure for a
blow that was inflicted by Heaven. This has been accepted
practice in all Jewish communities.

The *Bayit Hadash* clearly implies that it is incumbent upon the
patient to call upon God and also, eventually, to seek medical
advice; but it is forbidden to do neither.

In point of fact, this is also the opinion of Nachmanides. For in
his *Torat ha-Adam* he writes:

> Since the physician is permitted to heal, and healing is indeed a divine commandment, therefore the physician need have no fear of possible consequences. If he acts in accordance with his best judgment, healing is but the fulfillment of the divine commandment to heal.[5]

In fact, Nachmanides' words in his *Commentary on the Torah* and in *Torat ha-Adam* can be reconciled only if we assume that Nachmanides too holds that the physician is obligated to heal, whereas the patient has the right to prefer to rely entirely on God. However, if the patient has chosen not to do so, then he is obligated to seek medical treatment.

To come now to practical conduct, the Hazon Ish wrote:

> Personally I think that the natural striving to maintain one's health is an obligatory commandment. It is indeed one of the obligations contributing to the perfection of man's human form. . . . We have seen indeed that there were Talmudic sages who went to Gentile physicians and even to heretics in order to seek treatment. . . . *It is obligatory* to seek medical treatment for oneself, just as one is obligated to make an effort to treat his fellow man. Try, therefore, to overcome your natural inclinations, and follow the physician's instructions.[6]

Leading contemporary authorities agree that in our day, when there are no prophets, there is a universal consensus that it is obligatory to seek medical advice.[7]

From the *Posqim* we learn that a patient can be forced to follow the physician's instructions. Thus, Radbaz writes:

> You asked me to tell you the law concerning a patient whose medical treatment required desecrating the Sabbath, but who, being very pious, refused to have the Sabbath desecrated for his sake. . . .
>
> *Answer:* This is a pious fool, and he is punishable for so behaving. Generally speaking, I do not see any piety in such behavior, but rather the deliberate destruction of a soul. The patient must therefore be fed even against his will, or forced to do whatever else the physicians say to do. Otherwise it is tantamount to shedding blood. This is rather elementary.[8]

Similarly, the *Magen Abraham,* relying on the opinion of Radbaz, comments on the following decision in the *Shulhan Arukh:* "If one physician says that the treatment [which requires desecrating the Sabbath] is necessary, and another says it is not, then the Sabbath is to be desecrated." The *Magen Abraham* writes: "If the patient does not want to accept the treatment, it is to be forced upon him."[9]

In conclusion, a patient may be compelled to accept medical treatment, even against his will.

Compulsory Testing and Treatment

Members of High-Risk Groups

Our problem is not yet not solved, and this for two reasons:

1. When we are confronted, not with someone who is certainly sick and needs treatment but refuses to accept it, but rather with a high-risk group, only a small fraction of whose members would be found to be carriers of the etiological agent of the disease, is it permitted to enforce a test upon all members of the group in order to identify the minority who are carriers?
2. Is it permissible to make everyone in the group undergo a blood test against their will, an invasive procedure with some risk, albeit minimal?

It seems to me that the answer to both these questions is in the affirmative. It is permitted to make testing of high-risk groups mandatory, both for the benefit of the subjects themselves and for the benefit of the general public. Further, it is permitted to make blood tests mandatory, and the minimal risk involved should be disregarded.

First, we must define the halakhic meaning of the concept of high-risk group. Then we should apply the halakhic principle of epidemic to the members of a high-risk group. For example, if a city is affected by an epidemic, all its residents are regarded as a high-risk group whose members may contract the disease. Any segment of the population which is particularly susceptible to a disease, whether because of lifestyle (homosexuals) or a medical condition (hemophilia), is to be considered as present in an area of epidemic.

The Hatam Sofer was asked about fasting on Yom Kippur during a cholera epidemic. He took his cue from the discussions in which the *Posqim* ruled that a nursing mother is permitted to take food on Yom Kippur if her fasting would endanger the baby's life by reducing the vital milk supply; the mother is not to fast so as not to put the baby in a possible danger (*safeq piqquah nefesh*).[10] On this basis, the Hatam Sofer decided that "all the more is it permissible for a healthy person to take food [on Yom Kippur] if the fasting results in a possible danger: although this person is healthy at present and only the air is corrupt, still we have to be concerned about the possibility that he will be infected."[11]

Similarly, it is well known that during an epidemic of cholera, Rabbi Yisrael Salanter ate various foods in the presence of the whole congregation.[12] Again, the *Magen Abraham* writes: "Nowadays we do not fast at all during an epidemic, for we know from experience that when one does not eat and drink he may be affected by [illness-inducing] changes in the air."[13]

The Halakhah rules that if a patient says on Yom Kippur that he is not in need of food, but the physician says he is, then he is forcibly fed.[14] And since the *Posqim* have ruled that epidemics are to be equated with a state of acute disease, it follows that in a state of epidemic, too, we have to rule that "he is forcibly fed."

In the light of this, we conclude that in the case of an epidemic or of a high-risk group, compulsory medical treatment should be enforced.

For the Benefit of the Public

Up to this point we have discussed the halakhic sources according to which it is permitted to make it obligatory for members of groups with a high risk of contracting AIDS to be tested for their own benefit. Although the disease is as yet incurable, there is no doubt that timely intervention may lengthen the patient's life.

But compulsory testing may be enforced not only for the benefit of the members of the high-risk groups, but also because they are a danger to the public.

In the *Shulhan Arukh*, Rama ruled that "He who endangers the public, e.g., a forger in a place where the authorities are exacting, is considered a pursuer (*rodef*), and it is permissible to hand him over to the [Gentile] authorities."[15] It is also stated: "Therefore, a fetus which threatens the mother's life may be aborted, as it is, in effect, a pursuer, pursuing her with a view to killing her."[16] It is clear that the law of the pursuer (*rodef*) applies to anyone, even as blameless as a fetus, who endangers the life of others. In such situations it is permissible to destroy the pursuer or hand him over to the authorities.

It is known that high-risk groups endanger not only their own members, but also the general population. Therefore, even if they so endanger the general population without evil intent, their members are subsumable under the law of the pursuer. It should be noted that the law of the pursuer applies even in cases of doubt (*safeq rodef*), as, for example, in the case of a robber who may not have come with an intent to kill, but who is still considered a pursuer.[17]

It follows that members of high-risk groups must be compelled to undergo tests, on the grounds that they may be pursuers (*safeq rodefim*) who threaten the public welfare. According to the law, the pursued person must be saved, even at the cost of a physical injury to the pursuer if necessary. Certainly, taking a blood sample from a pursuer is less severe than saving a pursued person at the cost of a physical injury to the pursuer.

In addition, we may well apply here a principle established in the *Shulhan Arukh*,[18] according to which the city elders have the power to seize a person's property and even punish him physically if certain circumstances make this necessary or in order to check a threat (*migdar milta*); it is then permitted to "fine a violent person, excommunicate him, curse him in public, beat him, tear his hair out, and imprison him."[19] And surely no measure aiming to check a danger is of greater importance than one intended to prevent the contamination of many people by a deadly, incurable illness, when all that is required of the members of the high-risk group is a simple blood test.

Summary

Appropriate testing of high-risk groups is obligatory for three reasons:

1. Everyone is obligated to accept medical treatment if sick or in danger. Such treatment may be applied in a compulsory fashion.
2. High-risk groups are regarded as a *rodef*, i.e., pursuers of the general population.
3. The city elders may decree ad hoc regulations to curb a threat (*migdar milta*), even if they physically affect the inhabitants of the city. This surely applies in the case of AIDS, where the blood test required to identify the carriers of AIDS involves practically no danger.[20]

Notes

1. TB *Bava Qama* 85a.
2. TB *Berakhot* 60b.
3. Nachmanides, *Commentary on the Torah*, Lev. 26:11. Ed. H. D. Chavel (Jerusalem: Mosad Harav Kook, 1960), 2:186.
4. Rashba, *Responsa* 1:413; *Tur, Yoreh De'ah* 336; cf. *Beth Yosef.*
5. Nachmanides, *Torat ha-Adam, Sha'ar ha-Sakkanah.* Cf. H. D. Chavel, *Kitvey Rabbenu Moshe ben Nahman* (Jerusalem: Mosad Harav Kook, 1964), 2:43.
6. Hazon Ish, *Iggerot* 1:136, 138.
7. *Responsa Tziz Eliezer, Ramat Rahel* 20; *Responsa Yehaveh Da'at* 1:61.
8. Radbaz, *Responsa* 4:1139.
9. *Shulhan Arukh, Magen Abraham* on *Orah Hayyim* 328:6.
10. *Responsa Devar Shemu'el* 107.
11. Hatam Sofer, *Liqqutim* 23.
12. S. Y. Zevin, *Ha-Mo'adim ba-Halakhah* (Jerusalem, 1944, 1949), p. 83.
13. *Magen Avraham* 576:2; and cf. *Sedeh Hemed, Yom ha-Kippurim* 3.
14. *Shulhan Arukh*, 618.
15. *Hoshen Mishpat* 425:1.
16. *Hoshen Mishpat* 425:2.
17. *Sefer Me'irat Eynayim* 6.
18. *Hoshen Mishpat* 2.
19. *Sefer Me'irat 'Eynayim* 8.
20. This is not contradicted by the following passage from a responsum by Radbaz: "Amputation of even a non-vital limb can cause fatal bleeding. . . . I have seen a patient die from bleeding from small scratches made on his ear. This happened although there is no limb as slight as the ear" (Radbaz,

Responsa, pt. 3, 1052 [627]). It is, however, inconceivable that Radbaz was referring to a procedure similar to a modern blood test. See Dr. Levi's article "Kidney Transplantation and the Halakhah" (in Hebrew; *Noam* 14 [5731]: 308–324), where he wrote (p. 321): "Radbaz was referring to the state of medicine in his times, i.e., in the Middle Ages." And see also *Tziz Eliezer* 9:48, 10:25. I have discussed the issue at length in my article "Priorities in Lifesaving According to the Halakhah" (in Hebrew; *Diney Yisrael* 7 [5736]: 45–66).

Brit Milah and the Specter of AIDS (1989)

Alfred S. Cohen

One of the more frightening aspects of modern life is the specter of the AIDS epidemic, which has swept across continents like a whirlwind, bringing death and hysteria in its wake. At first considered an affliction which threatened only the fringes of society, AIDS has now come into its own as a threat to even the most clean-living and innocent persons. Retroactively, hospital patients who thought their lives had been saved by an emergency blood transfusion, or hemophiliacs who received blood treatments, or even nurses, doctors, and dentists have found out to their horror that not only have they become victims of the disease, but in addition, as carriers, they have unknowingly infected other innocent persons, family members, or friends.

No one, we are cautioned, can feel smugly secure that he or she is not at risk, that AIDS is of no concern. Consequently, we must re-examine some of our most common practices and consider whether modifications ought to be made, either as a precaution to stem the spread of AIDS or even as a measure of self-protection.[1] This is a particularly cogent question with reference to the performance of the *brit milah*, which is an almost universal practice among Jews. As we shall see, some of the halachic procedures attendant upon the *brit* may harbor tremendous dan-

113

gers not only for the baby or the *mohel* at any particular *brit*, but even for the entire Jewish community.

This study will examine the possible dangers and the halachic questions which need to be addressed in order to find resolution for what may prove to be a dilemma of epic proportions.

Although we are all familiar with the requirement of the Torah that all Jewish males receive a *brit*, we should not confuse this with the procedure loosely termed a "circumcision," or removal of the foreskin. Actually, *brit*, according to the halacha, is a more extensive procedure. The Mishnah in *Shabbat* 133a rules . . . עושין כל צרכי מילה בשבת מוהלין פורעין ומוצצין "On the Sabbath, we (must) perform all the requirements of *milah*: circumcision, *priah*, and *metzitza*." Thus, Jewish law apparently recognizes three parts to the *brit milah*—removal of the foreskin; *priah* which is tearing of the mucous membrane which lies under the foreskin; and *metzitza*, or "sucking out" the blood from the wound, for the purpose of cleansing the area and removing germs which might harm the infant.[2]

The traditional method of *metzitza* was—and is—accomplished by *metzitza be'peh*, whereby the *mohel* places his mouth over the wound and sucks out some blood. In light of the medical reality that one of the primary methods for transmitting the AIDS virus is by exchange of body fluids, particularly blood, there is great concern whether this *metzitza be'peh* is advisable or even permissible in our day and age.[3] Simply put, a *mohel* performs dozens, maybe hundreds of *milahs* a year, often upon children whose families he does not know at all. What if the father or mother of the baby had the AIDS infection, even for the most innocent of reasons, and the child was born harboring the virus? Potentially there may be great danger that the *mohel* may get infected. Is the *mohel* required to place himself in mortal danger? How integral a part of *milah* is *metzitza*, particularly *metzitza be'peh*? Or let us approach the matter from the other direction— what if the *mohel* is or, unbeknownst to himself, becomes a carrier of the virus? He could become another "Typhoid Mary," spreading the disease to hundreds of victims, unaware of what is happening. Are the parents obligated under Jewish law to place their son in such danger?

In order to answer these questions, we shall have to analyze a number of issues:

1.   What is the role which *metzitza* plays in the *brit milah?* Is it a therapeutic measure, essential for assuring proper healing? Or is it an integral part of the *milah* itself?

2.   How essential is *metzitza* specifically by mouth to satisfy the halachic fulfillment of the mitzvah of *brit milah?*

3.   Can or should the element of *pikuach nefesh* (mortal danger) obviate the requirement for *metzitza be'peh?*

4.   To what extent does medical opinion influence halachic decisions?

5.   *Metzitza be'peh* has been performed at all *brit milahs* for thousands of years. Is it permissible to relinquish a *minhag?* What is the power of a *minhag?*

In addressing these very serious questions, we are fortunate that we do not have to start *de novo*, for it is a topic which was at the center of a great deal of conflict and controversy during the nineteenth century, and there is an extensive body of halachic literature devoted to analysis of the question.[4] A major assault was undertaken by various Reform spokesmen in Germany during the course of the last century, attacking circumcision altogether as a vestigial barbaric ritual, an unworthy and unhealthy practice for people who considered themselves enlightened and rational. There were Reform "rabbis" and laymen who challenged the right of the Jewish *Gemeinde* (community organization) to force its members to circumcise their sons as a precondition for registering them as Jews. Even among those who did not seek to abolish circumcision entirely, there was nevertheless a widespread sentiment that *metzitza*—and certainly *be'peh!!*—was a disgusting, unsanitary, and totally unacceptable practice.

Consequently, many halachic authorities responded to the attacks on *brit milah*, in an effort to clarify and protect the traditional practices. But underlying all their careful analysis and explication is the awareness that, fundamentally, the "reformers" were mounting an attack on millennia of Jewish tradition in an attempt to break down the authority of Torah and tradition and replace it with their own concepts of a universal religion of "enlightened humanism." To their credit, the rabbis did not descend to the level of polemic and invective which was leveled at them, but chose to respond to the calumnies voiced against *milah* with reasoned arguments and careful explanation of the basis for the traditional practice.

The Maharam Schick took an active part in the controversy, for by the time he was writing he saw that the assault on *brit milah* was more than just an endeavor to improve the welfare of Jewish infants. He clearly understood that the true impetus for all the polemics was a challenge to the authority of the rabbis and, even more, a challenge to the supremacy of halacha, to the belief of *Torah miShamayim* (the Torah as being a Divine instrument). In his rulings he forbade a *mohel* from participating in a *brit milah* which did not include *metzitza be'peh*.[5] Moreover, he goes so far as to argue that possibly *metzitza be'peh* is on the level of *halacha leMoshe miSinai*—i.e., an express oral tradition dating back to Moshe Rabbenu—in which case, even if it could be argued that "Nature has changed," no change in the tradition could be countenanced.[6]

Furthermore, precisely because the challenge to traditional *brit milah* was perceived as an attack on the very heart of Judaism, he forbade even the slightest deviation from age-old practice.[7] היום אומרים לו עשה כך ולמחר כך, וחייב למסור נפשו "Because today they tell him to do this, and tomorrow they will tell him to do that—and therefore he is obligated to give his life [to uphold the principle that the laws of the Torah are inviolate]." In *Sanhedrin* 74 the Gemara teaches that when there is a general attack on Judaism, one must choose death rather than accept even so minor a change as modification of the traditional type of laces Jews used in their shoes. Maharam Schick considered the contemporary situation comparable in severity, and insisted that it is forbidden to budge an iota from previous tradition.

It is perhaps difficult to rely upon this aspect of the Maharam Schick's written response as a precedent in our own situation, for surely the current suggestion that some modification be introduced in *metzitza* is not coming at all from the camp of the irreligious or the anti-religious. Indeed, few but the most meticulous Jews are familiar with the practice of *metzitza be'peh*. Rather, rabbinic scholars and Orthodox medical professionals are raising the suggestion, and their sincere concern for the physical welfare of the Jewish community is not being seriously impugned. Fortunately, most of the rabbis who defended *brit* practices a century ago chose to buttress their opinion with careful and erudite halachic analyses of the purpose, importance, and rationale of *metzitza be'peh*. Their opinions are highly relevant to the present discussion.

The first point which needs to be clarified is the proper characterization of *metzitza*: what is its function? Usually, *metzitza* is seen as a measure instituted to assure the health and safety of the infant. Such is the view of R. Yaakov Ettlinger[8] relying on the Rambam.[9]

ואח"כ מוצץ את המילה עד שיצא הדם ממקומות הרחוקים כדי
שלא יבא לידי סכנה . . .

And afterwards, he [the *mohel*] sucks the *milah* until blood comes out [even] from the distant parts, so that [the child] will not be in any danger . . .

Following this reasoning, Rav Ettlinger refuses to sanction elimination of *metzitza be'peh*, which he concludes is the best way to draw blood even from the distant vessels.[10] His defense of *metzitza be'peh* was actually a counterattack on those who wanted to do away with the practice, which he maintained was an important safety measure.

Many rabbis contend that *metzitza* is a procedure mandated by the Gemara as a critical step in ensuring the cleanliness and promoting the healing of the incision. For that reason, the Gemara insisted that it be performed even on Shabbat (as *pikuach nefesh*), and instructed that any *mohel* who neglected this step was to be removed from his position.[11]

אמר רב פפי: האי אומנא דלא מייץ סכנה הוא ועברינן ליה
פשיטא מדקא מחלל עליה שבתא סכנה היא מהו דתימא . . .

However, reluctance to countenance any changes in the *metzitza* by mouth may arise from a different conception of that procedure: while it is true that it surely has a therapeutic purpose, there are some scholars who claim that *metzitza* is an integral part of the *brit milah* itself, not only an aid to healing. They interpret *metzitza* as fulfilling the obligation of *hatafat dam brit*, "letting the blood" for the purpose of establishing the covenant between G-d and the Jew.[12] This second interpretation arises from the somewhat ambiguous text of the Mishnah.[13]

עושין כל צרכי מילה בשבת, מוהלין פורעין ומוצצין ונותנין
עליה איספלנית וכמון.

On Shabbat, we do all that is necessary for the *milah*—we circumcise, we do *periah*, we suck out the blood, and we bandage the wound.

The question is where *metzitza* belongs in this list—is it part of the first group, the *milah* and *periah*, which are certainly the essence of the mitzvah, or does it go with the bandages which are clearly only necessary aids to maintain the infant's health?

Already in the days of the *Rishonim*, this question was taken up. The Ran[14] conjectures that were the *metzitza* only for medicinal purposes, the Mishnah would have termed it *refuah* (healing), rather than *tzorchai milah*, i.e., one of the necessities of the *milah*. ואפילו במציצה עד מה יש לעיין דכל דפרע הכי סיים צרכי המילה ודילמה המציצה יקריא רפואה ולא צורך מילה, וצ"ע. Obviously, resolution of this question is a major factor in determining whether modifications can be made in the *metzitza* process. If it is part of the *milah*, we have to follow exactly the criteria for correct *milah*; but if it was instituted to promote healing, and there are better or less dangerous methods available to promote healing, serious consideration ought to be given to these alternatives. Rav Asad, in his commentary on *Shulchan Aruch*,[15] points out a number of practical halachic differences which would arise from the latter reading of the Mishnah.

Nishtanah Hateva?

The nineteenth-century rabbinic defenders of *milah* also approached the subject from a different vantage: Let us assume that *metzitza* is not actually part of the *brit* itself but was instituted by the Gemara as an essential life-saving procedure. In that case, if one could demonstrate that lack of *metzitza* does not pose a mortal threat to the infant, it might be possible to make some change. That is not to say that the Gemara was mistaken when it declared *metzitza* vital. However, we do occasionally find our Sages concluding that *nishtanah hateva*, "Nature [of things or of people] has changed." When our own experiences directly negate an observed phenomenon in the Gemara, we are forced to conclude that the realities which they confronted were not the same as those we experience. Thus, we may posit that evidently things are not the same as they used to be.

Perhaps it would be possible to argue that albeit in talmudic times there was a danger to the child if *metzitza* were not performed by mouth, nowadays the medical reality is such that absence of *metzitza be'peh* does not pose a threat to the child's well-being. Such an argument need not be rejected on religious or procedural grounds, for eminent halachic authorities have employed a similar rationale for explaining other changes in Jewish law.

For example, the Gemara is of the opinion that a baby born in the eighth month is not a viable child;[16] technically, one does not violate the Sabbath to save such a child's life, since he cannot live anyway. But, as the Ramo[17] noted some four centuries ago,

> Many wonder at this [teaching of the Talmud that an eighth-month baby cannot live], for experience denies [the validity of their teaching]; therefore, we must say that nowadays *there has been a change in this matter* [emphasis added], and so in a number of situations.

> דאמרינן יולדת ל"ט אינה יולדת, כבר תמהו על זה רבים
> שהחוש מכחיש זה, אלא שאנו צריכים לאמר שעכשו נשתנה
> ואע"ג שהחוש העניין וכן הוא בכמה דברים.[18]

This was also the reasoning of Rav Yosef Karo, author of the *Shulchan Aruch*, in discussing another of the procedures of *brit milah*. It used to be the practice to wash the baby with warm water, both before and after the *brit*.[19] So vital was this measure considered for the baby's health that, if for some reason no warm water was available on Shabbat, it was even permissible to heat up water for this purpose.[20] Yet Rav Karo notes that nowadays this is not necessary—we see that babies are not washed with warm water, and nothing happens to them. Therefore, he concludes, it must be that *nishtanah hateva*, Nature has changed, and it is no longer an element of danger.[21]

We may not cavalierly declare, however, that any regulation which no longer appears necessary or rational should be abolished on the grounds that "Nature has changed." It is an argument that halachic experts are loath to employ, and one would hardly dare make such a declaration without ample precedent.

The *Tifereth Yisrael* undertakes to weigh the halachic validity of medical opinion; we cannot out of hand reject a medical statement which contradicts the Gemara, for, as we have seen, it is possible that matters have undergone a change since the time the Talmud was written. If it is necessary to conclude that *nishtanah hateva*, perhaps we will have to reach that conclusion. But ultimately, *Tifereth Yisrael* concludes that we cannot justify an argument of *nishtanah hateva* in this case. It has never been shown that sucking out the blood is *not* an important factor in the remarkable track record of *brit milah*, halachically performed, as a spectacularly safe procedure for thousands of years. Doctors readily admit that indeed there is some value to *metzitza*, and that it reduces swelling. Therefore, the nature of things has not really changed so much that we can reject the Talmud's evaluation. Consequently, he writes that *metzitza* must continue.[22]

Minhag

A further very strong consideration for continuing with *metzitza be'peh*, in the eyes of many rabbinic authorities, is the force of Jewish custom, a sacred *minhag* which has been observed for thousands of years. Not only is religious authority apt to be somewhat conservative when it comes to innovation, but the halacha itself grants tremendous significance to a custom; it is not to be taken lightly. This brings us to the next major question which we have to consider: how much weight does a *minhag* carry, under what circumstances may an alteration be made in age-old custom, and is such a change warranted by the present circumstances?

There is no question that in Jewish law, a custom attains great sanctity over time, sometimes even greater than that of a halacha. In *Yevamot* 115, the Gemara declares that even if Eliahu the Prophet himself were to appear and instruct us that we are mistaken in the way we perform a certain mitzvah, "we do not listen to him, since the people have already become accustomed [to do it a certain way . . .]." It is startling to discover that even when scholars realized that the community was following an incorrect custom, they were reluctant to effect alterations.[23] In *Taanit* 28b, we find Rav, the greatest rabbinic authority in all of Babylon, unwilling to stop the common custom of reciting *Hallel* on *Rosh Chodesh*, although, since the prayer was not warranted, they were reciting a *bracha* in vain, which according to many *poskim* is a transgression![24]

So strong is this sentiment that an accepted custom ought not be tampered with, even if it seems misguided, that Rambam penned the classical ruling, as follows:

והנהיג מנהג ופשט בכל ישראל ועמד בית דין אחר ורצה
לבטל אינו יכול לבטל עד שיהא גדול ממנו בחכמה ובמנין.

And if this custom was accepted and spread among all the Jews, and a later *Bet Din* wants to abolish [the custom], it may not do so unless it is greater [than the previous *Bet Din* which instituted the custom] in both wisdom and number.[25]

In light of the foregoing, it is understandable why the rabbis are so reluctant to countenance any tampering with the customary manner of performing *metzitza*. One could argue, however, that the Gemara never mentions *metzitza by mouth*. Although it is adamant about the importance of *metzitza*, it does not specify that it must be by mouth.

Perhaps based on this consideration, the community of Frankfurt-am-Main in 1885 published a pamphlet outlining the position of the Orthodox *Gemeinde* on this thorny question. Under the direction of Rabbi Samson Rafael Hirsch, the tiny embattled minority of Orthodox Jews had become a significant entity within the very bastion of Reform in Germany. While adhering strictly to the dictates of halacha, the committed Jews in Frankfurt nevertheless felt that they had to confront the reality of strong scientific objections to the traditional methods and respond to the denunciation of ancient *milah* practices as barbaric and atavistic.[26]

In the pamphlet, it was announced that hereafter all *milahs* performed in the *kehillah* would include *metzitza;* however, rather than exposing the open wound to direct contact with germs which might be present during oral suction, the *mohel* was to use a sort of glass tube, with an opening at the top, so that his mouth would not come into direct contact with the cut, nor would blood enter his mouth. The new directive sought to comply with the talmudic requirement of *metzitza* and even continue the ancient custom of *metzitza be'peh*, albeit with a slight modification which could nevertheless still be termed *metzitza be'peh*. Included in the pamphlet was a letter from R. Yitzchak Elchanan Spector, Rav of Kovno, expressing his approval of the new procedures. (In later years, acceptance was also to be forthcoming from Rabbi Chaim Berlin, Rabbi Chaim Soloveitchik, and Rabbi Aharon Kotler.)[27]

Nevertheless, there were and are *poskim* who reject the proposal as an unacceptable innovation, contrary to the established *minhag* which the Jewish people has observed for thousands of years. They insist that the halacha does require direct oral contact, pointing to the express statement of the Ramo and Maharil that the *mohel* must spit out the blood and that he has to rinse out his mouth before reciting the blessing.[28]

For those who follow the many *poskim* who approved the glass tube, it would seem to be an ideal solution for the AIDS problem, since according to many it satisfies the criterion of *metzitza* (and perhaps even *metzitza be'peh*), it does no violence to *minhag Yisrael*, and yet it conforms to the primary objective of our sages to promote greater opportunities for sanitary healing of the circumcision.

There is, furthermore, a very strong argument to be made to the effect that our sages were not reluctant to modify a custom if they perceived the innovation as an improvement. Interestingly, a classic example of this readiness to innovate occurs in connection with another part of the *milah* process—*periah*.

According to all halachic opinion, *periah* is part of *milah* as mandated by the Torah. Rambam[29] describes *periah* as ואח"כ פורעין את הקרום הרך שלמטה מן העור בצפורן ומחזירין לכאן ולכאן.

There is absolutely no ambiguity in his instructions: after the initial cut, the *mohel* should use his fingernail to tear the soft mucous membrane under the foreskin and roll it back on either side. The *Shulchan Aruch* likewise specifies this.[30] Yet R. Yaakov Emden, living in the eighteenth century, indicates that by his time it had long been the practice to perform *milah* and *periah* in one step instead of two. Furthermore, he cites sources to indicate that this change had been instituted at a much earlier date, perhaps even by the time of R. Hai Gaon, who died in the eleventh century! Nowhere is any objection recorded despite the fact that *periah* is unquestionably part of the *milah* itself, and if the procedure must be performed exactly as mandated since earliest times, this "innovation," one would think, should have evoked a storm of bitter criticism. There could have been ample grounds for objecting to a change in the *milah-periah*. The Midrash, extolling the wisdom and beauty of the human body which is uniquely constructed for the performance of mitzvot, notes that G-d gave people nails on their fingers so that they could perform the rituals of *melika* (a form of *shechita* of birds in the *Mikdash)* and *periah*. Nevertheless, when *mohelim* developed a more efficient method of performing *milah* and *periah* in one step, no objection was raised.

Perhaps we have to conclude, then, that the violent opposition to any modification of *metzitza* procedure in the nineteenth century arose not from the particulars of the suggested changes but rather from an awareness that the entire controversy was fundamentally a ruse by the enemies of Judaism to destroy the foundation of Torah observance. Thus, they were resisted absolutely, on ideological rather than on technical grounds. But in the absence of ideological bias, there may be times when modifications may be warranted or advisable.

Medical Opinion

The *brit milah* controversy in the last century highlighted a vexing problem in Jewish legal thinking, one which recurs in many areas of life, not just this one. How much validity should be given to scientific opinion when it comes to the formulation of normative Jewish practices? More specifically, how does the halacha react when scientific opinion seems to contradict talmudic principles?

Before we explore this topic, we must insert an *obiter dictum*: we discount altogether the scientific or medical opinions of people who do not believe in the Torah or who are advocates of a lifestyle contrary to Jewish thinking. As the *Tifereth Yisrael* wrote, in rejecting their contentions,

ואני מוסיף דאנו רואים היום דרופאי ישראל שהרוב שלהם . . .
ובזדון ליבם מיעצים להדיח בעניין אכילת איסורים.

> . . . for we see that the majority of Jewish doctors . . . out of the waywardness of their hearts advocate that [we] should eat forbidden [non-kosher] foods.[31]

However, in the present situation, the cautions voiced by immunologists about transmitting the AIDS virus are not directed specifically toward any Jewish practice; moreover, it is conscientious Orthodox medical professionals who are bringing to the fore their genuine concern that the traditional *milah* practice might inadvertently spread the disease.

Already in the days of the Gemara, we find that the rabbis did seek medical advice; however, it is difficult to gauge what credence they gave to medical opinion. In *Nidah*[32] we find the following account: R. Eliezer told about a woman who approached his father, R. Zadok, to find out what to do, for she was discharging "some sort of red pieces" (*k'min kelipot adumot*). R. Zadok asked the other Sages, and they asked the doctors, who responded that this woman must have some internal wound which is sloughing off these red pieces. They said, "Let her put the discharged pieces into water; if they dissolve, she is *tameh* (ritually impure)."

The Rosh[33] (in the early 14th century) pointed out the major difficulty with this passage—what is it coming to teach us? If the rabbis believed the doctors, why did they say to test the discharge? And if they were not prepared to believe the doctors, why ask their opinion? How then do we decide whether the Gemara felt that medical opinion has validity?

The Maharik,[34] also a *Rishon*, felt that the rabbis were indicating that they were prepared to follow the doctors' ruling.[35]

R. Yosef Karo, the great sage who wrote the digests which form the veritable foundation of Jewish law, seems to be prepared to rely on the medical profession. In *Bet Yosef*, he explains that since the doctors knew that such a discharge (as was described in the *Nidah* passage) cannot come from the uterus and of necessity has to be from the kidneys, we can rely on them.[36] Also, as we noted earlier, he was prepared to go along with the current medical thinking of his time which held that there was no need to wash a newborn baby with warm water before and after the *milah*, and therefore would not allow water to be heated up for this purpose on the Sabbath.[37]

But both rulings are challenged by the *Ramo*,[38] the Ashkenazi rabbi whose gloss on the *Shulchan Aruch* and *Bet Yosef* set the standard for Ashkenazi Jews. Commenting on the first case above, he writes

> And I am surprised at him, for it says in the Gemara that we do not rely on the doctors *alone* . . .

Apparently, he interprets the talmudic passage as indicating that the rabbis were interested to know the medical opinion but were not prepared to follow it slavishly; therefore, they advised the woman to perform a test to see whether the diagnosis was accurate.

Chatam Sofer, in the nineteenth century, is not prepared to give very much weight to medical opinion. However, he concedes that at the very least, the doctor's pronouncement should be enough to create a doubt in our mind. Thus, on Shabbat or Yom Tov, if the doctor declares that a patient's life is in danger, we follow his directions and transgress Shabbat or Yom Tov, not necessarily because we accept his word implicitly, but rather because his expert opinion is enough to engender a doubt, a *safek*. And in a situation of *safek pikuach nefesh*, the rule is that we take no chances and do whatever is recommended to save the patient's life.[39]

In a further explanation of his position, the *Chatam Sofer*[40] seeks to show that medical opinion is accepted by the halacha in a general sense only. But since it is not an exact science when it comes to issuing a ruling in any specific case, the rabbis should not rely on this general medical advice as binding. If they consider that the person for whom they have to make the ruling fits into the general category (*rov*), they may choose to rely on the doctors.[41] But, for example, in the case of an infant who has to undergo *brit milah*, the Gemara has a specific evaluation of the status of the child—the Gemara holds that there is a *chazaka* (prevailing condition) that all boys who are being circumcised are in mortal danger unless *metzitza* is performed. In such a case, the general medical opinion that germs are present and may cause infection cannot override the rabbinic certainty that if *metzitza* does not take place, the child is in danger of his life.

However, when the medical opinion (*rov*) does not contradict the prevailing reality (*chazaka*) as seen by our Sages, it seems prudent to take it into account. Thus, the glass tube or other methods of extracting blood from the wound would satisfy the dictates of halacha in a number of ways:

a. *Metzitza* is performed, assuring that blood is drawn from the wound, thus satisfying the criterion of the Gemara.
b. It is sanitary, thus avoiding the danger of contamination about which the medical profession warns.

To this writer, therefore, it appears that the solution offered by the Frankfurt community in the nineteenth century, and accepted by many leading *poskim*, would be an ideal solution to the problem posed by the AIDS epidemic. It ensures the child's safety by performing *metzitza*, which is a vital method of cleansing the wound, and it also guards against possible infection of either the child or the *mohel*. In short, it accords both with halachic requirements and medical guidelines.

Gloves

In a public statement criticizing the suggestion that *metzitza be'peh* be modified in order to avoid the spread of AIDS, Rabbi Menashe Klein[42] remarks that a far greater danger of spreading the disease exists in the *milah* itself, for it is not unusual for the *mohel* to nick himself accidentally during the procedure.

Although Rabbi Klein does not consider the advisability of the *mohel*'s using surgical gloves, that alternative seems obvious.

Dentists, nurses, lab technicians, and doctors now routinely wear gloves in the performance of mundane office procedures, for fear of inadvertently cutting themselves and coming into contact with the patient's blood or saliva. Is there any halachic reason why a *mohel*, too, should not protect himself by wearing gloves as he performs the *milah*?

In *Pesachim* 57a the Gemara criticizes a kohen who covered his hands with silk gloves while performing the Temple service. However, the disparagement arose because of his motivation— he wanted to keep his hands from getting soiled, an unworthy attitude towards the holy work in the *Bet Hamikdash*. Based on this talmudic text, the *Pitchei Teshuva*[43] rules that a *sofer* (scribe) may not write a *Sefer Torah* while he is wearing gloves.

However, if the motivation for wearing gloves were not personal fastidiousness but rather for protection or for sanitary reasons, it may be assumed that no objection would arise.[44]

Parental Choice

We are thankfully not yet at the point where AIDS imminently threatens the Jewish community, but were such dire eventuality to develop (G-d forbid), a case might be made for declaring that a father who nevertheless asks the *mohel* to perform direct *metzitza be'peh* would be placing his child in a potentially life-threatening situation. Does a father have the right to take that chance? May he declare himself willing to rely on thousands of years of precedent, trusting in the protection of G-d to save from harm those who are sincerely concerned to perform a mitzvah in the best possible way? Or would we say that he is forbidden to endanger his child for a standard of religious observance which is not required and which may even be contraindicated?

Actually, the father might have a precedent to draw upon. In the Gemara, Rav Poppa observes that although the rabbis had declared that on a very cloudy or windy day, no *brit milah* should take place (because the bad weather might be dangerous for the baby), nevertheless people do it all the time and nothing untoward occurs. He concludes that "since so many people do it, G-d watches out for the simple folk," and saves them from danger.[45]

The contention that when many people do something, even if it be dangerous, they will be saved from danger because "G-d watches over the simple" is indeed a rationale occasionally employed by halachists. For example, Rav Moshe Feinstein refused to declare smoking a forbidden habit although he conceded that much evidence pointed to its deleterious effect on health; he explained his refusal as based on the principle "since so many people do it, G-d watches out for the simple."[46]

It is only proper to question whether in the present circumstance, with AIDS being a very clear and present danger, anyone could legitimately argue that "many have done this" and "G-d has watched over them" because in truth, many people have engaged in behavior which is considered high-risk for contracting AIDS, and indeed, they have contracted it in ever-increasing numbers. G-d does not seem to be watching out for them at all. Even the most innocent victim of a blood transfusion has not been spared from the consequences of the AIDS virus. Under what pretext, then, could we venture the bravado to declare that "G-d will watch over the simple" in this instance?

Nevertheless, this rationale has been employed by a host of halachic decisors over the centuries, in a wide variety of situations, and some rabbis may choose to apply it here as well.

There is a further argument which could perhaps be offered to defend the position of those who want to proceed with the traditional *metzitza be'peh*, even if it is known to be dangerous and even if the ruling were rendered that it is not necessary. There is an impressive list of rabbis who, although in the minority, maintain that if an individual wants to be stricter than the law requires, he is permitted to do so, *even if it will result in his death!*[47] The Rambam is categorically opposed to this option, terming it a sinful act of suicide, and the majority of rabbinic decisors concur.[48] Nevertheless, there are some authorities who contend that an individual may exercise the option to be more strict (although he may not rule for the public that they must do so).[49]

Rabbi Dovid Cohen, in a lecture on the topic,[50] raised a further question. The *Avnei Nezer* maintains that an extra precaution is placed upon the rabbis lest a rabbinic ruling have the effect of obviating a mitzvah entirely. Should rabbinic authorities therefore have to take into consideration the eventuality that their ruling—that *metzitza be'peh* should not be performed as long as the threat of AIDS remains imminent—might result in the mitzvah being abandoned altogether? Or might they rely on those who, regardless of any rabbinic ruling, would adamantly continue to perform *metzitza be'peh*, reasoning that thereby the mitzvah will not be obliterated?

Suggested Remedies

What are the results of our investigation? Let us recapitulate the issues and problems we have discussed:

1. The Gemara considered *metzitza* a vital step to ensure the healthy recovery of the baby from the *milah*.
2. Challenges to Jewish practice based upon supposed scientific verities cannot be the determining factor in our religious lives. However, we are obligated by Jewish law to take into consideration the directives of the medical profession and take appropriate precautions.
3. Jewish thinking does not advocate closing our eyes and minds to medical or scientific realities, trusting that all will be well if we are sincere in our observance of mitzvot. The halacha will find ways to protect our welfare while adhering to the strict dictates of Jewish law.

A number of options lie before us, as individuals or as members of a community. First of all, of course, there is the option to do nothing, and to change nothing, trusting that *milah* will continue to prove beneficial for us and our children as it has for so many years. When the Romans threatened to kill any Jew who circumcised his son (in the Hadrianic persecutions of the second century), Jews nevertheless braved death to fulfill the mitzvah. Jews prevailed, while the Roman Empire has crumbled. The present danger, too, will pass.

Another remedy is suggested by Rabbi Menashe Klein in a public letter, wherein he adamantly defends *metzitza be'peh*. He proposes that the baby's blood can easily be tested for the presence of AIDS cells or antibodies prior to *milah*, and *mohelim* could be certified by their rabbis as having been tested free of AIDS contamination. These steps, he feels, would prevent the spread of the disease through *brit milah*. Although this is a very intelligent proposal, it might be exceedingly difficult to implement. Families might fear being labeled as AIDS carriers if their baby tested positive; there would be a great deal of pressure to suppress such findings, perhaps even to lie about them. In addition, it might be very difficult to get *mohelim* to agree to certification, and to assure that only "certified" *mohelim* be used. Moreover, the truth is that scientists just do not know enough about AIDS to be able to say with accuracy that a person is not incubating the virus. Our tests simply show whether the person already has the virus or antibodies in his blood, but are not able to determine whether they are yet to develop. Our knowledge is too scanty and our tests are not that reliable. Thus, this proposal may not actually offer an effective solution.

In the city of Baltimore, the rabbis and *mohelim* of the community have agreed on a plan which is admirably moderate, fair, and tolerant, while offering options which should win the approval of the most fearful parents or the most G-d-trusting ones.

The features of the Baltimore plan are as follows:[51]

a.   The plan does not go into effect unless all *mohelim* in the city agree to abide by its terms (which they have now all done).

b.   There will be no *metzitza be'peh* directly.

c.   *Metzitza* will be performed with a glass tube.

d.   If the father personally wants to perform *metzitza be'peh* for his own son, the *mohel* will instruct him how to do it.

e.   There is no objection to parents calling in a *mohel* from outside the city to perform the *milah*.

Other choices remain, and perhaps new ones will be suggested as we begin to know more about AIDS and how it is spread or can be prevented. In the meantime, the Frankfurt method, devised a century ago, still remains as an attractive alternative to the traditional *metzitza be'peh*. In the eyes of many leading *poskim*, it fully satisfies the requirements of halacha and retains our respect for Jewish traditions. At the same time, it seems to offer important safeguards both for the *mohel* and the baby; moreover, it may prove to be an important factor in preventing the spread of the disease within the Jewish community.

Until such time as there are more definitive pronouncements from our *poskim* on this topic, it seems to this author that discretion is the better part of valor. As it says in *Mishlei*, "The wise man has his eyes in his head."

Notes

1.   In recent years, it has become common practice in most mikvahs to place chlorine pellets in the water, to remove the danger of contracting AIDS or other communicable diseases.

2.   The Gemara considers the infants to be in mortal danger unless the blood is drawn out. For a more precise definition of this danger, see תפארת שדי חמד מערכה קונטרס המציצה and ספר זכרון ברית לראשונים and ישראל.

3.   AIDS is still a disease about which not enough is known. In an article in the *New York Times* on Friday, May 6, 1988, it was reported that preliminary research indicates that "human saliva contains substances which prevent" the AIDS virus from infecting white blood cells. Whether further tests will demonstrate that saliva is an effective barrier remains to be shown.

4.   שדי חמד, חלק ח, דף 281–236 .632–182 For a brief review of all the opinions, see משה בונם פירוטינסקי, ספר הברית (ניו-יורק תשל"ג), דף קפ"ה.

5.   שו"ת מהר"ם שיק יו"ד רמ"ד.

6.   He does not define how one determines what is a הלכה למשה מסיני.

7.   שו"ת מהר"ם שיק או"ח קנ"ב. As a student of the *Chatam Sofer*, Maharam Schick felt compelled to respond to a letter of the *Chatam Sofer* which had been published, declaring that *metzitza* is not an essential part of the *brit* and, if necessary, could be omitted. Maharam Schick writes that the letter was only discussing a case of הוראת שעה and was a case of the lesser of two evils, from which no precedent could be drawn.

8.   שו"ת בנין ציון א: כג, כד.

9.   הלכות מילה פרק ב הלכה ב.

10.   But see ספר הברית דף רי"ז, which cites the opinion of the Radvaz, who had a different understanding of this passage in the Rambam.

11.   שבת קל"ג.

12.   שו"ת מהר"ם שיק שם.

13.   משנה, שבת קל"ג.

14. חידושי הר"ן שבת קל"ב. Also cited in משנה ברורה. עיין מועדים וזמנים
של"א חלק ב ס' ק"מ בהג"ה אות ב.

15. יו"ד רנ"ח.

16. שבת קל"ה.

17. רמא, אבן העזר קנ"ו.

18. See also מגן אברהם קעג-א, קעט-ח; תוספות ע"ז כ"ד: ד"ה פרה; תוספות
מועד קטן י"א, ד"ה כוורא; צל"ח ברכות ט: תשובות חת"ם סופר קיא; חזון איש
אבן העזר י"ב אות ז.

19. משנה שבת פרק יט משנה ג.

20. שם.

21. However, the Ramo notes his disagreement with him on this point,
arguing that there has been no change.

22. תפארת ישראל, פרק י"א דמילה משנה ב אות ט"ו. This position was
approved also by R. Eliezer Horowitz, שו"ת יד אליעזר ס' נ"ה. In משנה ברורה,
דיותר טוב מציצה בפה ואפילו בשבת the Chafetz Chaim writes באור הלכה שלא א'
יש להתיר בספוג. I have also heard that in pre-war Vilna no mohel ever made
metzitza by mouth.

23. There are many other such instances recorded: באר שבע נ"ג considered the custom of kapparot on Erev Yom Kippur as wrong, similar to the forbidden דרכי אמורי. However, he would not change it. Similarly, the Bet Yosef
cites the opinion of the Ran, who considered that it was technically permissible
to chant the Megilla in translation, so that it could be understood by all, but
would not allow it because it would be a change in the custom. בית יוסף תר"ץ.

24. The text does add, however, that he would have stopped them were it
not for the fact that they omitted certain parts of the Hallel.

25. However, there is a distinction between the case cited by the Rambam
and the one we are dealing with: the Rambam discusses a regulation established by an official Bet Din, while it is difficult to know who instituted the custom of metzitza be'peh.

26. As reported in ספר הברית ר"כ.

27. שו"ת הר צבי רי"ד; פני הדור חלק ד קצ"ט; מהריץ חיות שכ"כ; ספר
הברית דף רכ"כ.

28. רמ"א יורה רעה רס"ה: א: מהריל הלכות מילה. ארי ליקוט תורה לך לך;
זהר כי תשא עמוד ק"ץ; שדי חמד דף 264.

29. הלכות מילה פרק ב הלכה ב.

30. יורה דעה רס"ד, ג.

31. תפארת ישראל, יומא פרק ח משנה ה.

32. נידה כב.

33. שו"ת ראש כלל ב סימן ח.

34. מהרי"ק שורש קנ"ט. This is in keeping with the halachic premise that
any "craftsman" can be trusted when speaking about a matter in his profession, since he would not want to jeopardize his reputation by lying. However,
the Maharam Schick (או"ח קנ"ב) writes that anyone who claims metzitza be'peh
is dangerous is just a "liar," for he himself had been a mohel for forty years and
had never seen any child have a bad experience. See also חת"ם סופר רעז, who

feels that we cannot rely on a phenomenon observed in the non-Jewish community to draw conclusions about the Jewish one.

For a complete study of the subject, see באר היטב יו"ד קפז-י"ז, חת"ם סופר, אבן העזר ב-ס"א, פתחי תשובה שם ס"ק-ל, תשובות פני יהושע לב-ד, משפט עוזיאל י"ד א-כ"ו, דעת כהן ק"מ, חכם צבי מ"ז, מנחת אליעזר חלק א-ג-ד-ה, הר צבי יו"ד קמט, שדי חמד מערכה יום כפור ג-ה.

35. When Rosh studied the passage, he apparently attributed the last sentence to the rabbis—i.e., they told the woman to make the test, in order to verify the medical diagnosis. But one could also attribute that last sentence to the doctors, who advised the rabbis to tell her to test their diagnosis. In other words, the doctors themselves might have wanted to confirm their diagnosis by means of a test. (תשובות עבודת הגרשוני כב See also חת"ם סופר יו"ד קע"ה about the advice of a non-Jewish doctor, and באור הלכה תרי"ח, who leaves the question of the reliability of a non-Jewish doctor's advice to the discretion of the rabbi.

36. יורה דעה קצ"א ד"ה כתב.

37. או"ח שלא.

38. יורה דעה קצא אות ד, או"ח שלא אות ב. Just how the Ramo differs in practical terms is not easy to understand. See his הגהות to the טור.

39. שו"ת חת"ם סופר אבן העזר ב: פ"ב. See also אגרות משה יו"ד ב-ס"ט.

40. שו"ת חת"ם סופר יו"ד. See further שדי חמד מערכה יום כפור נ אות כז קע"ה.

41. The Gemara, שבת קכח rules that for the first three days after a woman gives birth, she is not permitted to fast on Yom Kippur, and we violate the Sabbath for her. Rambam, in recording this law, adds "whether she says she needs it or even if she says she doesn't need it" (הלכות שבת פרק ב הלכה יג). The מגיד משנה records there a controversy among the rabbis, whether the Gemara posited the rule regardless of what the medical profession advises, or only if there is no medical opinion on the matter. He notes that Rambam was of the opinion that if the woman says she feels able to fast and the doctors also says that it is not necessary for her to transgress, then it should not be done. משנה ברורה ש"ל אות יא-יב rules similarly. See also באור הלכה יו"ד שכח"ח ד"ה ורופא.

42. In a public letter, dated 1988, Rabbi Menashe Klein of Brooklyn writes extensively refuting any arguments for elimination of *metzitza be'peh*, which he insists is a mitzvah, and anyone who does it will be protected. In the course of his argument, he notes that even if there is danger of transmission of disease, there is a far greater probability of its happening during the actual *brit*, for it often happens that the *mohel* nicks himself, and there could be an exchange of blood. If we accept the medical argument against *metzitza be'peh*, we would then have to be even more afraid to do *milah* altogether, and the mitzvah would have to be abandoned!

43. פתחי תשובה יו"ד רע"א אות י"ט.

44. ספר הברית דף קע"ט ע"ז.

45. יבמות עב.

46. ‏אגרות משה יו"ד ב' מ"ט‎. See further on this topic in the Ritva, as cited by ‏בית יוסף יו"ד רס"ב ד"ה גרסינן‎. The subject is also explored further in ‏ריטבא, יבמות יב; תרומת הדשן רי"א; יבמות ס"ד: אבן העזר סי"ט; חיים שאל חלק א' נ"ט‎.

47. In the mid-nineteenth century, there was a cholera epidemic, and many doctors warned that if people did not eat on Yom Kippur, they would be in great danger. *S'dei Chemed* reports that nevertheless, many rabbis did not permit people to eat, but no one died because he fasted. See ‏שדי חמד, מערכה‎ ‏מילה ב', אות ח', ר"ה ובקונטרוס; שדי חמד מערכה יום כפור ג', אות ד'‎. He implies that the *Chatam Sofer* ‏חלק ו כ"ג‎ agreed with those rabbis who allowed the people to fast and he seeks to infer from this that even if doctors declare it dangerous to make *metzitza be'peh*, nothing will happen to those who do it. However, a close reading of the *Chatam Sofer*'s actual responsum indicates that he opined that a person definitely should eat under those circumstances. For a complete discussion of whether a person should observe a mitzvah when there is danger to life, see ‏בית יוסף יו"ד קנ"א‎. See also my article "Potential Pikuach Nefesh: High-Risk Mitzvot," *Intercom,* a publication of the Association of Orthodox Jewish Scientists, April 1987, pp. 3–8.

48. ‏יחוה דעת ח"א מיסודי התורה ד'‎. See R. Ovadiah Yosef, ‏רמב"ם פרק ה' מיסודי התורה ד' ס"א‎.

49. ‏האלף לך שלמה שנ"ד‎.
‏רדב"ז, חלק ג' תמ"ד‎.
‏בית יוסף יורה דעה קמ"ז‎.

50. Annual Lupin Memorial Lecture, presented at Congregation Gvul Yaavetz Brooklyn, New York, on November 13, 1988.

51. Rabbi Heineman addressed the Association of Orthodox Jewish Scientists at their convention in June 1988 and outlined this plan.

Response to AIDS by the Jewish Community in the United States (1991)

כ/ג

Fred Rosner

The existence of Jewish patients with AIDS is well recognized. According to Dr. Harold Jaffe of the Centers for Disease Control in Atlanta, no one knows the actual number of Jews who are suffering from AIDS since such statistics are not recorded. Estimates range from several hundred to a thousand. In New York alone, more than forty members and friends of Congregation Beth Simchat Torah, the gay synagogue in Manhattan, have died.[1] The Chairman of the Board of that synagogue said at a meeting early in 1986 that he did not know even one rabbi he could call to counsel AIDS patients who asked him for help because of the fear and shame which make rabbis afraid to minister to such patients.[2] The gay synagogue in San Francisco, Shaar Zahav, has had several members of its congregation die of AIDS and has others who are now sick, according to Rabbi Yoel Kahn. The same is true of Washington's gay and lesbian synagogue, Bet Mishpachah.

Until recently, "the response of Jewish religious, communal, and organizational workers ran from paralyzing ambivalence to enlightened action."[3] Early in March 1986, three of Judaism's four religious branches joined with gay and lesbian Jewish groups and a variety of Jewish organizations including the Rabbinical Assembly (Conservative), the Union of American Hebrew Congregations (Reform) and the Association of Jewish Family and Children's Agencies in a task force to deal with the impact of AIDS on Jews.[4] The National Jewish AIDS Project, initiated by Daniel Najjar, its newly-named executive director, and Rabbi David Teutsch, executive director of the Federation of Reconstructionist Congregations and Havurot, became headquartered in Washington, D.C.[5] Absent from the leadership are representatives of the Orthodox Jewish community. The project

> will seek to provide pastoral care and counseling of patients and their families by rabbis and Jewish social workers; visitation of the sick by *bikur cholim* committees, delivery of kosher food to patients at home and in hospitals; and proper burial services from Jewish funeral homes. In addition, it will serve as an advocate of increased funding for hospice and home health care programs, and civil rights protection for persons with AIDS. . . . Special emphasis will be placed on outreach to both victims and their families.[6]

Temple Beth Torah in Dix Hills, New York, during the first week of March, 1986, sponsored a symposium on AIDS.[7] Rabbi Marc Gellman, spiritual leader of the synagogue and organizer of the symposium, said it was important for the synagogue to have hosted such a community discussion. "The synagogue should not be centered on religious activities as narrowly defined but as broadly defined," he said. "The priests in the Bible were involved in identifying infectious diseases. To think that we care only about holidays and prayer is wrong. This is a community issue and one the synagogue ought to address."

The Jewish Board of Family and Children's Services in Manhattan held an open conference on AIDS in December 1985 and began providing services to AIDS clients and their families, Jews and non-Jews.[8] New York's Federation of Jewish Philanthropies held a conference on February 6, 1986 dealing with the medical facts about AIDS and the resources being used to deal with it. On March 26, 1986, a conference was held at the Central Synagogue in Manhattan about AIDS and the special needs of the AIDS population. The following day, Federation's medical ethics committee, headed by Rabbi Moshe D. Tendler, conducted a symposium on the role of the family and society, as well as the religious implications of caring for AIDS victims. On May 7, 1986, yet another Federation-sponsored conference was held that dealt in part with the theological implications of the disease.

In Baltimore, Dr. Lucy Steinitz, the executive director of the Jewish Family Service, implemented policy and training for her caseworkers and volunteers to handle AIDS victims.[9] Peter Laqueur is a gay Jew who directed HERO, the Baltimore-based Health, Education, Resource Organization that acts as an AIDS clearing house, providing resources for medical, financial and counseling needs. Rabbi Mark Loeb of Baltimore's Beth El said of his congregants with sons who are gay: "It's a *mitzvah* to respond. We Jews, of all people, should understand pain and suffering. We need to be there for these people. We have a mandate to be there."[10] Rabbi Herman Neuberger of Baltimore's New Israel College noted that "no Jew in pain should be turned away. Being a homosexual is one thing, but having AIDS is after the fact and we as Jews need to administer care and counseling."

At its semi-annual meeting in White Plains, New York in December 1986, the Union of American Hebrew Congregations called on every arm of the Reform Jewish movement to educate its 1.25 million members about AIDS and urged its member congregations to help deal with the nation's escalating public health crisis. Rabbi Alexander Schindler, the Union's president, said to the 125 trustees:

> The challenge of our Jewish tradition is clear. Where there is illness and suffering, we must seek to comfort; where there is fear and prejudice, we must seek to dispel it with knowledge and education; where there is optimism and a commitment to life, we must seek to preserve the human spirit with hope and compassion.[11]

Schindler also reported on ways in which the organization was addressing the AIDS crisis.

Every Reform congregation in the U.S. and Canada received a packet of informational material about AIDS—including guidelines for counseling families of victims, names of local, regional and national support groups, hot lines and a suggested sermon—by early 1987.

Schindler announced that more than half of the organization's 13 regional offices will include workshops on AIDS at their forthcoming biennial meetings and that a cadre of rabbis and lay persons in each region would be trained to furnish counseling support and leadership on the subject.

Educational programs on the disease will be developed for use in the movement's adult education courses and for its youth division through its religious schools, summer camps and publications for young people, Schindler said.

He also told the trustees that AIDS would occupy a major place on the agendas of the spring convention of the Central Conference of American Rabbis (the Reform rabbinical organization) and the Union's fall biennial in Chicago, and so it did.

In Israel, the Health Ministry set up blood testing centers around the country to test for HIV antibodies. Although AIDS is not common in Israel, the testing of all donated blood ensures the lack of transmission of the disease to recipients of blood transfusions.

Notes

1. R. Elliott, "Jewish AIDS Care Program Launched," *Jewish Week*, March 7, 1986, pp. 5 and 46.

2. J. S. Deutsch, "Jews with AIDS: Community Faces a Tragic New Challenge," *Long Island Jewish World*, March 7–13, 1986, pp. 3, 13–14.

3. Ibid.

4. L. Cohler, "New National Group Formed to Help Jews Hit by AIDS," *Long Island Jewish World*, March 7–13, 1986, p. 10.

5. Elliott, op. cit.

6. Ibid.

7. S. Ain, "Health Expert: AIDS Spreading at Lower Rate," *Long Island Jewish World*, March 7–13, 1986, p. 12.

8. S. Ain, "N.Y. Jewish Groups Mobilizing to Meet AIDS Crisis," *Long Island Jewish World*, March 7–13, 1986, p. 12.

9. P. Jacobs, "AIDS, a Jewish Problem, Too," *Baltimore Jewish Times*, July 11, 1986, pp. 60–63.

10. Ibid.

11. "Reform Body Launches AIDS Program," *Jewish Week*, Dec. 12, 1986, p. 10.

Reform Responsa on AIDS

1. Jewish Reaction to Epidemics (AIDS) 1985

QUESTION: The current AIDS epidemic has led to much fear in various communities. Individuals afflicted with this disease have been removed from positions, ostracized socially, and their children excluded or segregated in schools. What has been the traditional approach of Judaism to such epidemics for which there is no known cure? (Rabbi G. Stern, New York, NY)

ANSWER: We must be concerned with the victims of AIDS as the disease is fatal; they need our compassion. We will not deal with the problems of sexual morality raised by AIDS in this responsum, but only with fear of the potential epidemic. The fear of the general population is understandable as little is known about the disease, its incubation period, or potential cure. Concern for both the individual and the community when a member is afflicted with a dangerous disease has been shown since Biblical times. The book of Leviticus contains detailed instructions of how a skin disease (*metzora*) is to be diagnosed and handled (Lev. 13). During the period of his illness the afflicted person was isolated. The priest who made the diagnosis examined that person after seven days, as well as subsequently. When the disease had come to an end, a complex ritual of purification was provided (Lev. 14 ff.). The precautions extended from the individual to the house in which he lived and it, too, was examined, and if necessary scraped and replastered and a ritual of purification was mandated.

Although we do not know the nature of the disease called *metzora* by the Bible, it was clearly contagious and led to vigorous efforts to isolate the individuals involved. These procedures were developed further by the Mishnah and Talmud. There are fourteen chapters in the *Mishnah Negaim* which deal with the subject in considerable detail.

Metzora was treated only from a ritual point of view by some authorities, so they did not apply the rules of non-Jews.[1] All contact with Jews who were afflicted was to be avoided. This included the sick person, his room, any food near him and even the air near the sick room.[2] Insects and flies which had contact with the diseased person were to be avoided.[3] For example, when the diseased person came to the *bet hamidrash* in order to study, he was separated from the other students by a wall which was to be "ten handbreadths high and four wide." It was also mandated that he enter the building first and leave it last.[4] These individuals were excluded from the community and usually lived outside of the cities (II Kings 7.3). If a man was afflicted by this illness his wife had a right to divorce and vice versa.[5] Those who suffered from such diseases were to avoid sexual intercourse.[6]

In the Talmudic period, individuals so afflicted were considered akin to the dead.[7] In the New Testament some such diseased individuals called to Jesus from a distance as they were obviously prohibited from approaching anyone in the community (Luke 17:12).

Discussions in the Talmud and the later responsa literature which dealt with other epidemic diseases usually were less drastic; they suggested that a fast be decreed as the pestilence was thought to be the result of community sins.[8] Jews in the Middle Ages like the rest of the population often fled whenever a plague or epidemic threatened. An epidemic existed if a smaller city suffered three deaths from a known disease on three consecutive days, or nine deaths in three days in a larger city (one which could provide 1500 young men as soldiers).[9]

The Jewish medical works of the seventeenth century contain regulations which govern epidemic diseases. As the garments of the sick were considered to provide a source of contagion, they were to be avoided until thoroughly aired. All drinking water was to be purified as a preventive against the epidemic.[10] Dr. Leon Elias Hirschel suggested a number of ways of fighting smallpox; they included quarantine and washing with vinegar by those who came in contact with the ill.[11] Israel Salanter took a humane and courageous approach to a cholera epidemic in Vilna during his lifetime as he urged the community to assist the victims.[12]

It is clear from all this that our forefathers sought to protect themselves through whatever ways were available from epidemics. The avenues of quarantine and flight were used.

In the current situation as we deal with AIDS, we should begin by following the advice of the medical community. The current medical opinion suggests that the disease is spread through sexual contact (homosexual or heterosexual), intimate contact and blood transfusions. Little is yet known, however, and there is no cure or preventive vaccine for AIDS, nor is anything known about its incubation period.

The fear and anxiety of employers, parents and others, therefore, can be understood. It is our duty to calm that fear and counteract the pressure of the media. In some instances quarantine or other measures may be appropriate, but they should not be undertaken lightly.

We should do whatever we can to minimize the suffering of the victims of this disease and help them and their families adjust to its tragic consequences. We should follow the advice of public health authorities in our attitude to employees and school-aged children.

2. Responsibility of an AIDS Carrier (1988)

QUESTION: An individual has been diagnosed as having AIDS. The testing has been positive, and there is little room for doubt, as he has developed some initial symptoms. Years may pass before other symptoms appear. It is currently estimated that at least 30 percent of carriers of the AIDS virus will be affected by the syndrome.

As a carrier he is also a transmitter of the syndrome; he is aware of the fact that the active stage of AIDS is fatal.

The young man in question insists on continuing to be sexually active and is careless about using preventive measures such as condoms. Would Judaism consider him a danger to society or, if married, to his wife? Would Judaism label his transmission of AIDS as murder? What are his responsibilities to society?

ANSWER: We sympathize with anyone stricken by this illness and must help him/her in every way possible. AIDS victims must be protected from needless discrimination, yet society must also protect itself from obvious dangers.

Let us view this question from two different perspectives. First, let us look at the matter of his sexual activity and Judaism's attitude toward this.

The question does not indicate whether the individual is homosexual or heterosexual, single or married. Let us initially assume that he is heterosexual, not married, and that his sexual activities are conducted with a number of different partners. Traditional and liberal Judaism have, of course, rejected promiscuous sexual activity, and we would reject his behavior on these grounds. In fact, the Talmud assumed that if a man had intercourse with a woman, it was intended to be serious and aimed at marriage.[13] There are many statements that prohibit sexual relations outside marriage.[14] This applies to both men and women. All unmarried individuals are to refrain from sexual intercourse.[15] Any male who violated this prohibition could be flogged;[16] more severe penalties were applied to females.

The efforts of traditional Judaism to segregate men and women sought to remove the temptations of sexual intercourse outside of marriage. Men and women were to be separated on all festive occasions in public places; a man was even prohibited from walking behind a woman for this reason, etc.[17] There are numerous similar citations in the Talmud, the codes, and the responsa literature. Despite this, such extramarital sexual relationships did exist and were sometimes defended as a human weakness.

Looser standards were tolerated in some ages, for example: in Judea in the Talmudic period,[18] in the Byzantine Empire, and in various Balkan lands in the last centuries.[19]

Yet consistent efforts were made to restrict sexual intercourse to marriage. In marriage, human sexuality was considered a positive experience. The tradition, of course, says much more on the subject.

We would therefore reject this man's promiscuous behavior and state that Judaism demands restraint and would punish violations when possible.

Now let us ask what our attitude would be if the individual in question is married. We must ask whether he can continue sexual relations with his wife. If he remains careless about his use of condoms he will probably transmit AIDS to his wife. No one is permitted to endanger the life of a fellow human being; one must die rather than endanger another human life.[20] As every source of *sakanat nefesh* must be removed,[21] this individual should *not* permit himself to continue sexual relations with his wife. This may ultimately provide grounds for divorce, which could be enforced by a *Beit Din*. A woman has always been able to seek a divorce if her husband was afflicted with leprosy.[22] or similar diseases. For that matter, she could seek it if her husband engaged in a new field which was noxious to her (e.g., tanning of hides).[23] Certainly, if the danger is great, as is the case with AIDS, grounds for divorce exist, though we would discourage a divorce and encourage the wife to support her husband in this difficult period when he needs her help. The couple must, however, refrain from intercourse or use stringent precautions.

We should also view this situation from the point of view of transmitting a fatal disease. Traditional literature, from the biblical period onward, has dealt with dangerous contagious diseases through quarantine.[24] In biblical times every effort was made to isolate the individual and to protect the general society from the dangerous but not fatal *tzara'at*. In this instance we are dealing with a fatal disease the effects of which are felt over many years. This means that a false sense of security may be given to both the carrier and the recipient. It also remains possible for the carrier to hide his condition from the recipient in the early stages of the symptoms.

We are aware of the tragic consequences for the individual who has AIDS and must sympathize with his/her plight. Every possible support and help must be extended to such an individual. His/her right to work and to function in a normal manner in our society must be protected. Yet such a respect for individual rights cannot be permitted to endanger others through reckless behavior.

Our present knowledge of AIDS and the lack of any cure or immunization lead us to view as a murderer a known carrier who is aware of his/her condition and engages in sexual relations without the regular use of condoms.[25] This must be made absolutely clear to such individuals; society can demand that they refrain from all sexual activity or protect their partners with great care. Such partners must be adequately warned.

If such demands cannot be met, then society must protect itself by isolating such individuals and utilizing every means at its disposal to protect the remainder of society as no individual has the right to endanger the life of another. It is incumbent on all members of society to protect themselves against such reckless and dangerous behavior.

Walter Jacob, *Chair*
CCAR Responsa Committee

3. Responsibility of an AIDS Carrier: A Communication (1989)

In the Spring 1988 issue of the *Journal of Reform Judaism*, there appeared a responsum on the question of "Responsibility of an AIDS Carrier" (above, p. 141–149). Rabbi [Walter] Jacob, writing for the CCAR Responsa Committee, walked a fine line as he attempted both to show compassion for the sufferer and to recognize his own "responsibilities to society." I respectfully submit the following for additional consideration.

Over the past year and a half, I have been involved in several seminars on AIDS at Yale–New Haven Hospital. Recently, our congregation sponsored an ecumenical "Service of Healing" for

AIDS and ARC (AIDS Related Complex) patients and their families. Soon after this service, I received a call from a local physician. He had a patient, a young Chasid, who suffered from
hemophilia. Because of the necessary and frequent blood transfusions he had received over the years, the Chasid had been
tested for AIDS and was found to be HIV-positive. The physician was told that a *shiduch* had been arranged with a young
woman in another community and that the Chasid would marry
despite the fact that he was HIV-positive—"It was in God's
hands." The *mitzvah* of *periya ureviya* was absolute.

The physician asked two questions of me. First, what Jewish
law, if any, forbids such deception? Secondly, as a "fallen away
Jew," what was his (the physician's) duty to his patient and to
the young woman?

Because of the young man's religious perspective, I sought
out an Orthodox authority whose answer could be used by the
physician in future conversations with the patient. In a letter to
the Agudath Israel of America, I asked for a halachic responsum
to this young man.

Within a matter of days, I received a phone call from an Agudath Israel attorney, who also introduced himself as having *semi-
cha*. He told me that Agudath Israel could not (or would not) put
a responsum in writing because of the complex legal issues that
could be involved. He also felt that time was of the utmost
importance. He assured me, however, that he had queried six
experts (*posekim acharonim*) and they were unanimous in their
position.

First, as to the young man's plans to marry an unsuspecting
woman, the marriage itself would be null and void. In fact, one
posek suggested that even if the girl had known and agreed to
the marriage, it would not be allowed. The *mitzvah* of *periya ureviya* is precluded in this case by the groom's illness, since it
would, by its very nature, jeopardize any issue of the marriage.

Secondly, the attempt to deceive the bride amounted to an
avera. The potential groom was in fact a *rodef*, a pursuer whose
actions threatened the life of another, and, according to the Talmud,[26] to act in such a way could be construed as a capital
offense.

Thirdly, as to the physician's responsibility vis-a-vis the young woman, the *posekim* quoted the biblical admonition: "*Lo ta'amod at dam re'echa*" (Lev. 19:16). Further, *pikuach nefesh* requires the physician to intercede on behalf of another human being.

One *posek* referred to the Maimonidean Medical Oath, to wit:: "Thy eternal providence has appointed me to watch over the life and health of Thy creatures." The ability to help save a human being is tantamount to the obligation of doing so. That ability (in this case the knowledge of the HIV-test result) was a divine gift, perhaps for this very purpose.

I was surprised by the directness of Agudath Israel's responses, which I think should help further clarify the responsibilities of an AIDS carrier.

Herbert N. Brockman
Congregation Mishkan Israel
Hamden, Connecticut

4. Tahara and AIDS (1990)

QUESTION: At the present time the funeral director of the local Jewish funeral home refuses to permit *tahara* for AIDS victims. Are there circumstances under which *tahara* may be withheld (for example, dangerous infectious disease), or should we insist that he treat AIDS victims like all other dead?

ANSWER: The fact that this question is asked at all indicates the progress of modern medicine in removing the danger of most infectious diseases. Through most of our long history the grave danger of plagues and major epidemics was, of course, recognized even while the danger of infectious diseases was not. Special precautions were occasionally initiated during major epidemics, but those who died from any disease were treated alike and were provided with the same preparation before burial. In fact, crises like epidemics and plagues led to the creation of new burial societies and to renewed devotion to proper burial.[27] Special burial preparations were made only for those who were murdered or those who died in childbirth.[28]

There was, of course, considerable discussion in the rabbinic literature about the reaction to plagues. Flight from the affected areas was encouraged.[29] Solomon ben Simon Duran[30] approached the whole matter from a philosophical point of view and asked whether flight would be successful if an individual had already been destined for death. Isaac Luria devoted an entire chapter to the question.[31] There is a large number of responsa that deal with contagious diseases and ways to escape epidemics.[32] Flight was the principal remedy.

Those who were not fortunate enough to escape and died were to be buried in the appropriate manner. It might be possible to throw quicklime on the grave in order to avoid the spread of the plague.[33] Furthermore, the laws of mourning could be modified or suspended in these sad times.[34]

Although these modifications were readily undertaken, the basic rites of burial were followed as closely as possible. In other words, there is no doubt that in times of mass deaths, when a large proportion of the community had fled, some normal honors accorded to the dead were no longer possible. Yet there was no question about *tahara* or any matter connected with burial or the preparation for burial.

The local funeral director is obligated to perform *tahara* and to treat AIDS victims as all other dead in accordance with local custom and the specific wishes of the family. The funeral director would be encouraged to take all possible precautions to prevent infection by AIDS.

Walter Jacob, *Chair*
CCAR Responsa Committee

5. *Testing for HIV (1990)*

SHE'ELAH: I have been informed that the Syrian-Sephardi Rabbinical Association of Brooklyn passed a resolution that they will not officiate at any marriage until they have received documentation attesting to the fact that both parties have undergone testing for the human immunodeficiency virus (HIV). Should Reform rabbis make the same requirement? There seems to be a parallel to the resolution we passed on Tay-Sachs disease. (Rabbi Alexander M. Schindler, UAHC, New York)

TESHUVAH:

I. Halakhic Precedents

The primary role of someone officiating at a marriage *(mesadder kiddushin,* usually a rabbi)[35] is to make sure that a valid marriage is being entered into.

Circumstances may arise under which the rabbi would refuse to officiate. A well-known example is that of an inebriated groom who is unable to enter into a legal obligation. In such an instance the rabbi's judgment not to proceed with the ceremony is not contested.[36] Since there is halakhic precedent for rabbinic refusal *under certain circumstances,* we must now ask whether the unwillingness of the couple or one of the partners to be tested for HIV would constitute a cogent reason for the rabbi's unwillingness to officiate.

1. The rule that he/she would likely invoke is that of *pikku'ach nefesh,* the protection of life. Our tradition is firm in holding that, when *pikku'ach nefesh* is at stake, all mitzvot may be disregarded save bloodshed, idolatry and sexual transgressions *(gilluy arayot).*[37] One who is too concerned with halakhic propriety when life is endangered is regarded as a shedder of blood.[38]

The officiating rabbi has also another (though implied) role, namely, to prevent a transgression from being committed. In the case of HIV and the possibility that it will develop into the acquired immune deficiency syndrome (AIDS), a disease for which there is presently no cure, the command that stands in danger of being violated would be "Do not stand idly by the blood of your neighbor."[39] R. Jacob Breisch derives from this Torah proscription a specific instruction to physicians to inform the healthy party to a prospective marriage that the other partner is afflicted by a dangerous disease.[40] In instances of this kind the person carrying it might be considered a *rodef* (literally "pursuer")[41] who, albeit unintentionally, threatens the life of an innocent person.[42]

Can R. Breisch's reasoning guide us in the question before us? Would the rabbi, like the doctor, be considered guilty of standing idly by the blood of the couple, should it turn out that indeed one of them is infected with HIV?

We believe that the precedent to which R. Breisch addressed himself is not operative here. The physician has *actual knowledge* of the presence of a dangerous disease and therefore is required to disclose that fact, while the rabbi has no knowledge of the couple's personal exposure and knows only that many people in society carry the virus. There is a gulf between knowledge of the actual and fear of the potential.

It is worth noting, however, that the mere potential of a life-threatening situation was dealt with by the Hatam Sofer (Rabbi Moses Schreiber/Sofer) some 150 years ago. There was a severe outbreak of cholera in Europe, and physicians had warned that fasting on Yom Kippur might make people more susceptible to the disease. In view of this medical judgment the rabbi, who was Europe's leading halakhist, permitted the consumption of food in quantities sufficient to prevent Jews from being overly weakened. Even though the violation of a direct prohibition was at issue, R. Sofer's permission (*hetteir*) functioned as a prophylactic, to prevent people from becoming ill.[43] But not all authorities agreed, and some urged their congregants to observe the fast if at all possible. Still others promoted the idea of shortening the services.[44]

As in R. Breisch's ruling, we feel that the precedent of the Hatam Sofer (if we were to agree with him) is not applicable to our case. For his *hetteir* was advisory and not compelling. People were free to disregard it.

More recently, this question, with specific reference to AIDS, was addressed by Rabbi Shelomo Deichowsky, a rabbinical court judge in Israel.[45] He asserts that, while the community is entitled to issue rulings (*takkanot*) in order to protect itself from various dangers, he would agree to particular measures for at-risk persons (*kevutzot sikkun*). He does not suggest that the general population be required to undergo testing.

In sum, we have not found the kind of precedent that would speak unequivocally to the *she'elah* before us. But before we go further it is well to look at an entirely different aspect, which is the right to privacy.

2. Actually, while it is not proper to speak of "rights" under Jewish law, there are numerous instances when it treats of obligations which in other legal systems might be termed "rights." Thus, a homeowner may take action to protect his household against the prying eyes of neighbors;[46] or we may note the Torah's prohibition of gossip (rekhilut).[47] Tradition goes so far as to proclaim that someone who shames another in public has no place in the world to come.[48]

R. Eliezer Waldenberg has applied the issue of halbanat panim (making someone blanch with embarrassment) to a medical situation and ruled that, while a physician may ordinarily bring medical students to a patient's bed, this should not be done when it causes halbanat panim.[49]

Thus, while the right to privacy as such has no direct precedent in Jewish law, its objective—to safeguard the dignity of the individual—clearly has. In the case of AIDS, an illness surrounded by popular superstitions and anxieties, the possibility of having test results revealed (to public bodies or others) poses a definite threat to privacy and arouses fears of unwarranted disclosure and slander.

In sum, for reasons set out above in (1) and (2), halakhic precedents would lead us to view compulsory testing with caution.

II. Further Considerations

What other consideration might then be brought to bear on the issue, and further, what additional guidelines might we obtain from precedents in the literature of the Reform movement?

1. The first that comes to mind is a resolution of the Central Conference of American Rabbis (CCAR) which, in 1975, called on its members "to urge those couples seeking their officiating at marriage ceremonies to undergo screening for Tay-Sachs and other genetic diseases which afflict Jews to a significant degree."[50]

That resolution, however, is not fully applicable to our case. For one, Tay-Sachs is a disease which afflicts Ashkenazic Jews in significant proportions, while HIV/AIDS have no such specific identification with Jews. Secondly, the rabbis were called upon to *urge, but not require,* couples to undergo testing. Hence, we cannot take this resolution to guide us in our answer.

2. Various jurisdictions have instituted certain pre-marriage requirements (e.g., Wassermann tests), and rabbis in such states have an obligation to await the issuance of a license before they officiate. In Illinois, beginning January 1, 1988, all marriage applicants *have been required by law to prove that they have been tested for the presence of HIV antibodies,* and that the test results have been communicated to a government health agency as well as to both parties in the proposed marriage. But that law is operative only in Illinois, and since we have been asked whether rabbis should undertake a similar program for their people, we should look at the results of the Illinois statute.

In the year since the law was instituted, only 26 people out of 155,458 marriage license applicants were found to test positive. Either the incidence of HIV is very low in the state or, more likely, the figures are skewed, in that they do not take into account those prospective marriage partners who did not want to be tested and therefore went outside the state for their marriage. Under the circumstances, C. Kelly, a member of the Illinois Department of Public Health, judged the whole procedure not to be cost-effective.[51]

In the question before us, the Illinois experience would lead us to conclude—

a.   that if we were to require marriage applicants to be tested for HIV, those who believe themselves at risk would search out another rabbi or functionary who does not make such a requirement;

b.   that we, as rabbis, have little reason to believe that, were we to require tests, we would be more effective than the state of Illinois.

3. Since the rabbi would request only that tests be *taken,* not that their results be *revealed* to him/her,[52] the couple's privacy may not at first sight appear to have been invaded. Yet a closer

look at the interplay of private concerns and public policy does give us second thoughts.

In many places the process of HIV testing itself has serious social consequences. For instance, physicians or institutions that do the testing may be obligated to register any positive finding with a government health agency, as is the case in Illinois. In our present climate of gross and unwarranted discrimination even against persons *suspected* of infection, the very process of testing is laden with the danger of divulging private information—a danger which is enhanced by the potential accessibility of our electronic storage systems as well as by the still error-prone testing for the virus—there being both "false negative" and "false positive" results. For these reasons many persons who fear that they might have the HIV hesitate to submit themselves to testing.

Despite the fact that California provides the strongest protection for the preservation of confidentiality, an examination of pre-1989 legal cases indicates a serious erosion of medical privacy for HIV infected persons.[53] A rabbinic either/or requirement might therefore lead the couple to do something that will indeed expose them to social and psychological injury and make the rabbi an unwitting party thereto.

4. In the presence of HIV/AIDS we are faced with deep "social fears," and therefore protection of the dignity of the individual must be a paramount concern.[54] This is a matter to which the CCAR has addressed itself repeatedly. In 1954 it said: "No free society can long survive if its citizens are encouraged or permitted to inform indiscriminately on one another."[55]

While that resolution spoke to the concerns of the McCarthy era in the United States, its message remains valid even when the informing arises from medical reports. In 1955 the CCAR further stated: "The pivotal problem which confronts us today remains that of the proper balance between individual freedom and national security. Our Conference has spoken in clear and forthright terms on the subject."[56]

To be sure, HIV is different from the concern for national security referred to in the resolution, but the whole fabric of protection for the individual is affected when a portion of the citizenry is unduly exposed to state interference. Both in the 1950's and 1990's, the individual must remain on guard against the incursion of the collective, and the rabbi should not by his/her actions diminish the protected realm of those who wish to arrange for their marriage.

5. But should we not consider the spread of AIDS a veritable plague which would sweep aside these considerations? To put it differently, does the interest of the community not require us to override our obligations to the couple and their right to privacy?

While, with regard to the spread of AIDS, the term epidemic is frequently used, it does not describe an illness against which the population cannot protect itself adequately. Rather, there are high-risk groups which are indeed gravely exposed and require urgent attention, but the majority of the population continues to experience low-prevalence exposure.[57]

6. We frequently deal with couples who are already living together and are now contemplating marriage because they wish to have children. Our responsibility should therefore be to help safeguard the health of such future offspring, and we should warn the couple that, since HIV is transmissible *in utero*, testing prior to marriage is highly advisable.

7. The question may also be asked whether Reform rabbis, who do not function in a judicial capacity, would go beyond their duties when they decide that the particular couple is not fit to be married. This kind of judgment is in any case highly problematic and should not be exercised unless very particular circumstances obtain.

8. Finally, we should also note the special characteristics of Syrian-Sephardi communities, such as the one referred to in the *she'elah*. They are tightly knit, family-like groups with strong internal controls, which observe, for instance, a stringent ban against conversions for the sake of marriage.[58] We lack that kind of disciplinary control, even if we were to contemplate exercising it.

III. Conclusion

While halakhic precedents are inconclusive or cautionary regarding a rabbinic requirement to undergo pre-marital testing,

other considerations would lead us to counsel against such procedure.

Though we have every regard for the seriousness of AIDS and
are committed to extending our compassionate care to those
afflicted by it, we cannot state that its spread is of pandemic proportions, nor do the results of compulsory testing in Illinois convince us that rabbinic action would be successful and wise.

Advising couples about testing is one thing and is encouraged;
requiring them to undergo it is not, at least at this time. Should
conditions change we would be open to reconsider our position.

(Postscript 1995: The above responsum was written in the
winter of 5750/1989–90, and the best data then available led us
to our conclusion. Since then, the disease has taken on epidemic
dimensions in certain parts of Africa, while in North America
and other Western nations it remains confined to high-risk portions of the population. A review of up-to-date literature led
Prof. Joseph Adelson of the University of Michigan to state in
1995 that AIDS will not touch most heterosexuals.[59])

CCAR Responsa Committee
W. Gunther Plaut, *Chair*
Mark Washofsky, *Vice Chair*
Solomon B. Freehof, *Honorary Chair*
Judith Zabarenko Abrams
Richard A. Block
A. Stanley Dreyfus
Walter Jacob
Peter S. Knobel
Dow Marrnur
Richard Rosenthal
Louis J. Sigel
Moshe Zeiner

Notes

1. M. Neg. 3:1.
2. San. 76b; *Lev. Rabba* 17:3.
3. Ket. 77b.
4. M. Neg. 13:12.
5. M. Ket. 7:9.

6. Ket. 77b.
7. Ned. 64b.
8. M. Avot 5:12; Ta'anit 3:4, 19b.
9. Ta'anit 21b.
10. Tobiah Hakohen, *Ma'aseh Tuvyah* (Frankfurt am Main, 1707), in Max Grunwald's *Die Hygiene der Juden* (Dresden, 1912), p. 262.
11. "Abhandlung von den Vorbauungs- und Vorbereitungsmitteln bei den Pocken" (Berlin, 1770), in ibid., p. 265.
12. D. Katz, *Tenu'at Hamusar* (Tel Aviv, 1946), vol. 1, pp. 156 ff.
13. "*Ein adam oseh be'ilato be'ilat zenut,*" Yev. 107a; Ket. 83a, Git. 81b.
14. Prov. 6:29, 32; Lev. 19:29, 20:10; Tos. 14, etc.
15. Pes. 113a ff., Shab 152a, San. 107a, Ket. 10a, etc.
16. Ket. 10a.
17. *Yad,* Hil. Yom Tov 6:21.
18. Ket. 7b.
19. L. Epstein, *Sex Laws and Customs in Judaism* (New York, 1948), p. 128.
20. San. 60b ff.; A.Z. 43b, 54a; Ket. 33b; Shabbat 149a; *Sefer Hamitzvot,* Lo Ta'aseh, nos. 2 ff., 10, 14; *Shulchan Aruch,* Yoreh De'a 157:1.
21. Deut. 4:9, 4:15; Ber. 32b, B.K. 91b; *Yad,* Hil. Rotzeach Ushemirat Hanefesh 11:4–5, Hil. Shevu'ot 5.7, Hil. Chovel Umazik 5:1.
22. M. Ned. 11:12.
23. M. Ket. 8:9.
24. See "Jewish Reaction to Epidemics—AIDS," *Contemporary American Reform Responsa* (New York, 1987), no. 82. (In this volume, above, p. 139–141.)
25. For a discussion of condoms and other birth-control devices, see the lengthy responsum by J. Z. Lauterbach in W. Jacob (ed.), *American Reform Responsa* (New York, 1983), pp. 485 ff.
26. TB. San. 72b.
27. I. Abrahams, *Jewish Life in the Middle Ages* (Philadelphia, 1911), pp. 355 ff.
28. For a summary, see J. J. Greenwald, *Kol Bo al Avelut* (New York, 1965), pp. 49 ff., and *Sedei Chemed* IV (Avelut, no. 141).
29. *Shulchan Aruch,* Yoreh De'a 116:5 and commentaries; see also J. Preuss, *Biblical and Talmudic Medicine* (New York, 1978), pp. 151 ff.
30. *Responsa,* Maharil, no. 195.
31. *Yam Shel Shelomo* 6:26.
32. H. J. Zimmels, *Magicians, Theologians, and Doctors* (London, 1952), pp. 99 ff. and 193 ff.
33. *Shulchan Aruch,* Yoreh De'a, Pitchei Teshuva; Jacob Reischer, *Shevut Ya'akov,* II, no. 97.
34. *Shulchan Aruch,* Yoreh De'a 374:11, and commentaries.
35. The emergence of the rabbi as the primary *mesadder kiddushin* has been set forth in a *teshuvah* written by R. Solomon B. Freehof and issued for the CCAR Responsa Committee; see *CCAR Yearbook* 65 (1955): 85–88.

36. *Peri Megadim,* Orach Hayyim 573, Mishbetzet Hazahav, n. 11 (refusal because of inebriation); *Resp. Minchat Yitzhak* I 10 (refusal to officiate for an apostate); *Resp. HaRambam,* Blau, n. 347 (refusal until groom, who is not known in the community, proves he is unmarried or divorces his present wife).

We might here also mention Mishnah Ketubot 7:10, which states that men with certain skin diseases are compelled to divorce their wives. The Mishnah speaks of *shehin,* which is variously understood as a skin disease in general, or leprosy, or boils. It is also identified as the *holi tsarfati,* or syphilis; see Be'er Hetev to *Shulhan Arukh,* Even Ha-Ezer 154. The mishnaic obligation to divorce would appear to apply to a man having AIDS and thereby give the rabbi (who knows at the time of marriage of the presence of the disease) reason to refuse officiating.

37. B.T., Yoma 85b, Sanhedrin 74a; Rambam, *Yad,* Yesodey HaTorah 5; *Shulhan Arukh,* Yoreh De'ah 157.

38. *Shulhan Arukh,* Orach Hayyim 328:2.

39. Leviticus 19:16.

40 *Helkat Ya'akov* 3:136, on the basis of his reading of Rambam's *Hilkhot Rotze'ach* 1:14.

41. The Halakhah has made this term a legal concept, and someone so designated may be killed before he/she can kill. [In 1995 the designation by some rabbis of Yitzhak Rabin as a *rodef* became the subject of widespread controversy after the Prime Minister was assassinated. It was believed that this designation moved the killer to commit the deed.]

42. See Bi'ur HaGera on *Shulhan Arukh,* Hoshen Mishpat 425, n. 11

43. *Resp. Hatam Sofer* 6, n. 23.

44. See *Matteh Efrayim,* chap. 618, Elef Ha-Magen.

45. *Assia* (published by the Falk Schlesinger Institute at the Shaare Zedek Medical Center in Jerusalem), January 1989, pp. 28–32. (In this volume, above, p. 105–112.)

46. *Hezek re'iyah* is treated in Mishnah, Baba Batra 3:7; Rambam, *Yad,* Hilkhot Shekhenim 5; *Shulhan Arukh,* Hoshen Mishpat 154.

47. Lev. 19:16; the Rambam lists three types in an ascending order of severity, the worst offense being the spreading of news which, though true, is damaging to someone else's reputation (*Yad,* Hilkhot De'ot 7:2).

48. B.T., Baba Metsi'a 59a; Rambam, *Yad,* De'ot 6:8.

49. *Resp. Tsits Eliezer,* vol. 13, n. 81, sec. 2.

50. *CCAR Yearbook* 85 (1975): 79.

51. Fifth International Conference on AIDS, *Abstracts* (Montreal, June 1989), p. 68.

52. We have not been asked what consequences might ensue for the rabbi should a positive test result come to his/her attention. This would raise additional halakhic as well as general legal questions. A responsum on aspects of this issue was published by Walter Jacob, *Contemporary American Reform Responsa* (New York, 1987), no. 5, "Confidential Information."

53. *Abstracts* (see above, n. 51), p. 945; report by Clint Hockenberry, AIDS Legal Referral Panel, San Francisco.

54. Ibid., p. 967; lecture by C. Aredondo, Spanish Ministry of Health.

55. *CCAR Yearbook* 64 (1954): 54.

56. Ibid. 65 (1955): 65.

57. Ida Onorato, Centers for Disease Control Atlanta, *Abstracts* (above, n. 51), p. 78. See further *Population Reports,* Series L (Population Information Program, Johns Hopkins University, Sept. 1989), especially p. 4. The report covers North America as well as other areas. A survey of HIV prevalence on university campuses in the U.S. produced a rate of 0.2% (Helene Gayle, Centers for Disease Control; *Abstracts,* p. 79). Even among homosexuals and bisexuals, reported AIDS cases are leveling in selected metropolitan areas, including New York, Los Angeles and San Francisco (Ruth Berkelman, Centers for Disease Control, ibid., p. 66). AIDS researcher Dr. Catherine Hankins reported that in Montreal about one in every 400 women giving birth is HIV infected. "The rates are higher than we predicted and they reflect the increasing role that heterosexual transmission of HIV is playing in Quebec" (*Globe and Mail,* Toronto, Nov. 17, 1989). The infection rate quoted, though higher than that reported in San Francisco, is still only 0.25%, which can hardly be termed epidemic. See also the latest report of the (U.S.) Federal Centers for Disease Control, reported in the *New York Times,* January 4, 1990.

58. See Moshe Zemer, "The Rabbinic Ban on Conversions in Argentina," *Judaism,* Winter 1988, pp. 84–96.

59. *Commentary,* July 1995, pp. 26–30. He bases himself primarily on E. O. Laumann a.o., *The Social Organization of Sexuality: Sexual Practices in the United States* (Chicago: University of Chicago Press, 1994).

Statements on AIDS by Jewish Organizations in the United States

׳ק

Resolutions Passed by
The United Synagogue of Conservative Judaism

1. Resolution Passed in 1987: AIDS

WHEREAS, in the Bible and in the Talmud the Jew is mandated to maintain the health of the body, noting that the body itself is a reflection of the divine, and legislation was promulgated early on in the history of the Jewish people to treat illnesses and to curb plagues; and

WHEREAS, in the recent past a plague has emerged threatening the well-being of the human community through the contagious disease of Acquired Immune Deficiency Syndrome (AIDS);

BE IT THEREFORE RESOLVED that our affiliated congregations seek to heighten the consciousness about this disease and to convey whatever information is available for its prevention; and

BE IT THEREFORE RESOLVED that we call upon the public media, namely newspapers, radio networks and television stations, to disseminate information about the preventive measures that must be taken in order to control this affliction.

2. Resolution Passed in 1989

WHEREAS, The United States of America, Canada as well as the rest of the world is currently experiencing one of the most devastating public health crisis faced in modern times, Acquired Immune Deficiency Syndrome (AIDS), a disease which has the possibility of devastating society; and

WHEREAS, Confusion, ignorance and denial are among the most common responses to the AIDS epidemic; and

WHEREAS, Jewish law, custom and tradition clearly mandate all Jews to maintain the health of the body, noting that, according to the Bible itself, the body is divine, and legislation was promulgated early in the history of the Jewish people to treat illnesses and to curb plagues; and

WHEREAS, The religious community has a clear responsibility to help create awareness and sensibility to the crisis of AIDS by utilizing the public media, newspapers, radio networks and television stations to disseminate information about the preventative measures that must be taken in order to control this affliction;

THEREFORE, BE IT RESOLVED, That the UNITED SYNAGOGUE OF CONSERVATIVE JUDAISM calls upon all of its affiliated congregations to affirm the Mitzvah of Pikuach Nefesh (the saving of lives) by instituting comprehensive, effective and age-appropriate educational programs about preventing transmission of the AIDS virus; and

BE IT FURTHER RESOLVED, That the UNITED SYNAGOGUE OF CONSERVATIVE JUDAISM affirms that those infected with the AIDS virus must be protected from all forms of illegal discrimination, such as discriminatory housing, employment, health care delivery services and synagogue services; and

BE IT FURTHER RESOLVED, That no congregation within UNITED SYNAGOGUE OF CONSERVATIVE JUDAISM shall exclude Persons With AIDS (PWA) from synagogue life; and that the Jewish Theological Seminary of America be urged to train Rabbis and other Jewish professionals to deal with and counsel Persons With AIDS.

·3. Resolution Passed in 1991

WHEREAS, the world is currently experiencing one of the most devastating public health crises faced in modern times, Acquired Immune Deficiency Syndrome (AIDS), a disease which has the possibility of destroying society as we know it; · and

WHEREAS, confusion, ignorance and denial are among the most common responses to the AIDS epidemic; and

WHEREAS, Jewish law, custom and tradition clearly mandate all Jews to maintain the health of the body, noting that, according to the Bible itself, the body is divine, and legislation was promulgated early in the history of the Jewish people to treat illnesses and curb plagues;

NOW, THEREFORE, BE IT RESOLVED that the UNITED SYNAGOGUE OF CONSERVATIVE JUDAISM calls upon all of its affiliated congregations to affirm the mitzvah of *pikuah nefesh* (the saving of lives) by instituting comprehensive, effective, and age-appropriate educational programs about preventing transmission of the AIDS virus; and

BE IT FURTHER RESOLVED that in the spirit of *bikkur holim* (visiting the sick), the UNITED SYNAGOGUE OF CONSERVATIVE JUDAISM calls upon all of its congregations to reach out to individuals infected with the AIDS virus, their families and their friends by providing acceptance, comfort, counseling, and sympathetic and empathic listening; and

BE IT FURTHER RESOLVED that the UNITED SYNAGOGUE OF CONSERVATIVE JUDAISM affirms that those infected with the AIDS virus must be protected from all forms of illegal discrimination such as discriminatory housing, employment, health care delivery services and synagogue services; and

BE IT FURTHER RESOLVED that no congregation within UNITED SYNAGOGUE OF CONSERVATIVE JUDAISM shall exclude persons with AIDS (PWAs) from synagogue life; and that the Jewish Theological Seminary of America be urged to train rabbis, cantors, and other Jewish professionals to deal with and counsel people with AIDS and their families.

Resolutions of the Rabbinical Assembly Plenum Conventions

1. Resolution Passed at the 1987 Convention: AIDS

WHEREAS thousands of people are now experiencing the terror of an epidemic outbreak of Acquired Immune Deficiency Syndrome—(AIDS); and

WHEREAS there is at present no cure for AIDS; and

WHEREAS this illness is an occasion of great physical pain for the afflicted individual as well as a trial of great psychic suffering, legal disabilities, and economic stress upon the patient, as well as his or her family, friends and community; and

WHEREAS the Jewish tradition has always placed its highest priority upon the notion of *pikuah nefesh*, attending to the health-care needs of individuals, and to the accompanying needs of the patients;

THEREFORE, BE IT RESOLVED that we, the members of The Rabbinical Assembly, in convention assembled, demonstrate our compassion to all those affected: patients, parents, partners, families and friends; and declare that all mitzvot making manifest Judaism's love of all human beings and Judaism's compassion for the sick appertain hereto with full force, including such areas as *bikkur holim*; and decry all unjust discrimination in such areas as medical attention, housing, insurance and education; and

BE IT FURTHER RESOLVED that The Rabbinical Assembly charge its Social Justice Committee to assist in this gathering of appropriate information; and

BE IT FURTHER RESOLVED that The Rabbinical Assembly call upon the media, private corporations, government agencies, and other public communication networks to fully educate the community at large about the nature of this fatal illness, about safety measures to prevent acquiring or transmitting the disease, and about caring for AIDS patients with dignity.

2. Resolution Passed at the 1991 Convention

Resolution on Medical Ethics and the AIDS Epidemic

WHEREAS AIDS has reached epidemic proportions throughout the world and requires enormous commitments of medical treatment to those living with the disease, and

WHEREAS many people, even including clergy, frequently reflect a common societal tendency to feel ambivalent or fearful towards those persons living with AIDS, even as to the amelioration of their suffering, and

WHEREAS health-caregivers are themselves not immune to this mindset, and have often, in all too many cases, declined to serve patients who are HIV-positive,

THEREFORE BE IT RESOLVED that the Rabbinical Assembly does hereby express its conviction that the refusal by a rabbi to minister to a person with AIDS or to the family of such a person is a *Hillul HaShem*, and that the refusal of health-caregivers similarly to minister to such a patient is a violation of their professional duty.

Resolution: AIDS & Health-Caregivers

WHEREAS health-care professionals have in many cases themselves become victims of AIDS and other life-threatening contagious diseases, and have, perhaps understandably but nonetheless questionably, chosen to hide their condition out of fear of exposure,

THEREFORE BE IT RESOLVED that the Rabbinical Assembly does urge HIV-infected health-caregivers and health-caregivers infected with any life-threatening contagious disease to reveal their medical status to any patient to whom they attend.

The Reform Movement

ఈ

Resolutions Passed by the Central Conference of
American Rabbis (CCAR)

1. Resolution Adopted by the Annual Convention
of the CCAR in 1986: AIDS

WHEREAS AIDS, Acquired Immune Deficiency Syndrome, has become a major health problem in North America and throughout the world, and

WHEREAS the horror of this as-yet incurable disease is exacerbated by ignorance of the means of transmission of the disease, and

WHEREAS the United States Supreme Court has recently ruled permitting American businesses to discriminate against persons who have tested positive for HTLV-III virus and patients who have developed AIDS, and

WHEREAS the United States Justice Department has recently ruled the persons who have tested positive for the HTLV-III virus and those who have developed AIDS are not protected by existing federal statutes concerning persons with handicaps,

THEREFORE BE IT RESOLVED that 1. The Central Conference of American Rabbis extends its praise and support to the Union of American Hebrew Congregations, which has boldly undertaken pioneering initiatives in both policy and program in regard to AIDS, in creating a national task force on AIDS. We urge our members to support the UAHC in its activities in this area. 2. We call upon our members to make known to their various congregations and other constituencies those facts that are known and that will become known about AIDS. As a particularly urgent matter, we urge publicity concerning the fact that giving blood to blood banks involves NO risk of contracting AIDS. 3. We further call upon our members and our congregations to extend warm and loving support to those persons who contract AIDS and to their families, exercising the mitzvah of *bikkur cholim*, especially in those cases that so often have elicited rejection rather than care. 4. We wholly reject the suggestion that has been offered by some, that AIDS may be understood as a special punishment visited by God on a particular class of sinners. AIDS is a viral disease, and, as such, follows natural laws. The difficult theological problem of suffering must be solved for all cases, not dealt with in only those areas where prejudice is substituted for reason or love. 5. We call upon our national governments to include all individuals who have tested positive for the HTLV-III virus infection or who have developed AIDS within the scope of existing federal, state, and local statutes protecting the rights of the handicapped. We call upon our national governments to provide adequate financial and scientific resources to work toward developing a cure for this disease.

2. Resolution Adopted by the Executive Board of the CCAR in 1990: AIDS

WHEREAS, the Central Conference of American Rabbis resolved in 1986 to support education and ethical action programs about AIDS, and

WHEREAS, the UAHC Task Force on AIDS has done exceptional work in recent years, and

WHEREAS, the Israeli AIDS Task Force has also done exceptional work,

THEREFORE, BE IT RESOLVED, that we call upon all of the constituencies which we serve to create and implement an AIDS policy that would respond to the needs of their personnel, as well as their members.

BE IT FURTHER RESOLVED, that we call upon all of our colleagues and staff people, who serve with them, e.g., cantors, educators, administrators, et al, to become fully educated regarding every aspect of the AIDS epidemic and its impact upon society, and to facilitate AIDS education programs within their work places and elsewhere in the communities in which they reside.

BE IT FURTHER RESOLVED, that we call upon all of our colleagues to assist in the formation and implementation of local and regional AIDS Interfaith Councils and to work with all clergy in the fields of AIDS education and outreach.

BE IT FURTHER RESOLVED, that we call upon our colleagues to take all necessary steps so that each community in which they serve has in place outreach to Jewish persons with AIDS and to their loved ones; i.e., pastoral care, funding for those in need, alternative medical care systems, etc.

BE IT FURTHER RESOLVED, that we call upon our colleagues to express their concern in those instances when health insurance coverage is withheld from persons suffering from AIDS inasmuch as serious illness and impoverishment are linked together so profoundly.

BE IT FURTHER RESOLVED, that we call upon the government of the United States to increase funding for AIDS research and the distribution of any and all drugs which have proven to be effective in treating persons who show evidence that they are HIV-infected and who are financially or otherwise incapable of purchasing these medications.

BE IT FURTHER RESOLVED, that in accord with the biblical dictum, "Neither shall you stand idly by the blood of your neighbor," we urge all health care professionals, including those in the psychiatric, psychological and nursing professions, to reaffirm their own sense of obligation to those suffering from AIDS and to their families.

)

Index

Note: Not included are names of Mishnaic and Talmudic rabbis, as well as names of authorities used only to designate halakhic works (thus Maimonides and Nahmanides are included, but not Rif, Tur, Rosh, etc.). The spelling of names follows their first occurrence in the book.

169

Acknowledgments

 צ׳ה

The texts gathered in this volume have all been published previously and are reprinted here with the kind permission of the respective copyright holders.

Lord Immanuel Jakobovits, "Only a Moral Revolution Can Contain This Scourge" appeared in *The Times* (London), 27 December 1986, p. 20.

"Memorandum on AIDS" and "Halachic Perspectives on AIDS" appeared in *Assia: Jewish Medical Ethics* 2, no. 1 (January 1991): 3–8. The three texts are reprinted with the kind permission of Rabbi Lord Jakobovits.

Barry Freundel, "AIDS: A Traditional Response," first appeared in *Jewish Action*, Winter 5747 (1986–87): 48–57. It is reprinted with the kind permission of Rabbi Barry Freundel.

Fred Rosner, "AIDS: A Jewish View," was first published in *Journal of Halacha and Contemporary Society* 13 (Spring 1987/ Pesach 5747): 21–41 and subsequently reprinted in F. Rosner, *Modern Medicine and Jewish Ethics*, 2nd revised and augmented edition (Hoboken, N.J.: Ktav Publishing House, New York: Yeshiva University Press, 1991), pp. 49–63. It is reprinted here with the kind permission of Dr. Fred Rosner.

Abraham Steinberg, "AIDS: Jewish Perspectives," first appeared in Hebrew as "AIDS—Hebetim Refu'iyim, Musariyim, we-Hilkhatiyim," *Assia* 47–48 (vol. 12, nos. 3–4)

(Kislev 5750/1990): 18–30. The English translation of a slightly modified text appeared in *Medicine and Jewish Law*, edited by Fred Rosner, vol. 2 (Northvale, N.J.: Jason Aronson, 1993), pp. 89–102, and is reprinted here with the kind permission of Professor A. Steinberg and Dr. Fred Rosner.

David Novak, "The Problem of AIDS in a Jewish Perspective," was first published in *Frontiers of Jewish Thought*, edited by Steven T. Katz (Washington, D.C.: B'nai B'rith Books, 1992), pp. 141–156, and was reprinted in David Novak, *Jewish Social Ethics* (Oxford: Oxford University Press, 1992), pp. 104–117. It is reprinted here with the kind permission of Professor David Novak.

Benjamin Freedman, "An Analysis of Some Social Issues Related to HIV Disease from the Perspective of Jewish Law and Values," first appeared in the *Journal of Clinical Ethics* 1, no. 1 (Spring 1990): 45–49 and is reprinted with the kind permission of Professor Benjamin Freedman and the *Journal of Clinical Ethics* (copyright 1990).

Shlomo Deichowsky, "Compulsory Testing and Treatment for AIDS," first appeared in Hebrew as "Kefiyat Bediqah we-Tippul—Hebetim Hilkhatiyim al Mahalat ha'AIDS'," *Assia* 45–46 (vol. 12, nos. 1–2) (Tevet 5749): 28–33. An abridged English translation appeared as "Compulsory Testing and Therapy for AIDS," *Assia: Jewish Medical Ethics* 2, no. 2 (May 1995): 10–12. The translation, which has been thoroughly revised for the present volume by Gad Freudenthal, appears here with the kind permission of Professor M. Halperin, director of the Dr. Falk Schlesinger Institute for Medical-Halakhic Research at the Shaare Zedek Medical Center Jerusalem, publisher of *Assia: Jewish Medical Ethics*.

Alfred S. Cohen, "Brit Milah and the Specter of AIDS," first appeared in *Journal of Halacha and Contemporary Society* 17 (Pesach 5749/Spring 1989): 93–115. It is reprinted with the kind permission of the *Journal of Halacha and Contemporary Society*.

Fred Rosner, "Response to AIDS by the Jewish Community in the United States," is a section of Fred Rosner, "The Acquired Immunodeficiency Syndrome (AIDS): Jewish Perspectives," which appeared in *Jewish Values in Health and Medicine*, edited by

Levi Meier (Lanham: University Press of America, 1991), pp. 171—184, on pp. 174–177. It is reprinted with the kind permission of Dr. Fred Rosner.

Reform Responsa: "Jewish Reaction to Epidemics (AIDS)" is reprinted from *Contemporary American Reform Responsa*, edited by Walter Jacob (New York: Central Conference of American Rabbis, 5747/1987), pp. 136–138, with the kind permission of the CCAR Press. "Responsibility of an AIDS Carrier" is reprinted from the *Journal of Reform Judaism* 35, no. 2 (Spring 1988): 81–83, with the kind permission of the CCAR Press, publisher of the *Journal of Reform Judaism*. "Responsibility of an AIDS Carrier (A Communication)" is reprinted from the *Journal of Reform Judaism* 36, no. 1 (Winter 1989): 89–90, with the kind permission of the CCAR Press, publisher of the *Journal of Reform Judaism*. "*Tahara* and AIDS" is reprinted from the *Journal of Reform Judaism* 37, no. 2 (Spring 1990): 65–66, with the kind permission of the CCAR Press, publisher of the *Journal of Reform Judaism*. "Testing for HIV" is reprinted from the *Journal of Reform Judaism* 37, no. 3) (Summer 1990): 59–66 (with slight modifications by Rabbi W. Gunther Plaut, chairman of the CCAR Responsa Committee, which authored the responsum) and is reprinted with the kind permission of the CCAR Press, publisher of the *Journal of Reform Judaism*.

Statements by Jewish Organizations: 1. (I) The resolutions passed by the United Synagogue of Conservative Judaism are reprinted with the kind permission of the United Synagogue of Conservative Judaism. (II) The resolutions passed by the Rabbinical Assembly are reproduced with the kind permission of the Rabbinical Assembly. 2. The resolutions passed by the Central Conference of American Rabbis and by the Executive Board of the CCAR are reprinted with the kind permission of the CCAR Press.